Dedicated to those suffering from mystery symptoms

Have courage, and keep asking questions. You *can* be healed.

What is **TILT**?

Toxicant

Induced

Loss of

Tolerance

Contents

Preface

The story I am sharing is true and presented here just as I experienced it. Please understand the information in this book is not *medically* proven, but it does accurately represent my son's mystery illness and his healing. Names and locations have been changed to protect us from potential retribution from my son's previous employer.

For ten years my youngest child (let's call him Clint) tried to get well the traditional way, only to become sicker. I know that what we did, with our backs up against a wall, worked.

Having written the book in a nonfiction format initially, and recovered from the opinion of my attorney, it remains important for me to provide this information to the world. I very much hope you are so amazed by this journey that you'll continue to read until the very end.

Hello. Let's say my name is Peggy Marshall—that is, Peggy Marshall writing as Margaret Starr.

Introduction

I have been told I am a warrior. As I begin to write this book, I wonder where this came from. As I close my eyes to connect with my deep inner thoughts, I remember.

I was young. Was I in junior high or high school? I cannot remember. I am just beginning to piece the memory into place like a huge puzzle with its pieces dumped onto the floor. I wonder—will all 2,500 pieces of my puzzle still be there and match the beautiful picture on the box lid when I'm finished? Or will some pieces be lost forever from their connection of the perfect-picture world?

I know I am young. Too young for such a responsibility. I accept the gift in fear. After all, what can I say to my great-aunt when she asks me to carry her earthly spirit in my heart before she quietly slips into the unknown world of death? I have only a few minutes to spend with her before she will be gone. I just lie as still as I can in the darkness of my bedroom on this unexpected and scary night.

I am sleeping. Am I dreaming? Whose face is that in the dark? I open my eyes, and the image stays. It's my great-aunt Martha from my dad's side of the family. She's standing over my bed. She seems so serious and sad. I want to reach out to her. I cannot.

She holds out her arm, like it's a signal for me to be patient. She has something to say, and it must be important.

I wait. Scared. Not moving. I don't want to wake my sister, just a few feet away. This is my special time, and I don't want to share. No matter how scared I am.

"Peggy," my aunt says, "I must go now. My time has come, and I am leaving you. I'm sorry. I will miss you the most. I have always felt closest to you. You are a strong person. Life is not easy. You were born to be a protector. This is your destiny."

I listen and try to understand what she means. She must go? Go where? On vacation? I want to go. I understand this is not what she is talking about.

Aunt Martha continues. "I am giving you my spirit. I will always be in you. I will give you strength. Any time you have large doubt and confusion, I will be there. Just look within yourself, and you will find my strength to guide you through the rough roads in life."

I want to ask her questions. I need to know what she means and what I am supposed to do with this information. Can I tell anyone? Why can't she come and help me in person when I need her?

She tells me she has to go. She says it is time. "Goodbye."

I am quickly brought into awareness as the telephone rings downstairs; I can hear my father running down the hall to answer it. It is dark; it's the middle of the night.

"Who died?" I hear him ask. "How long ago? What happened? She was only in her fifties." His conversation continues, but I can't listen. I have way too much to think about. "What just happened?"

He hangs up and makes more phone calls. I already know who has died. Her angel came to tell me. She is with me to this day.

One

Way Back When

Long before large chemical companies dominated our existence, the eagles tried to tell us what DDT was doing to them. "Whwee! Whwee! Stop the chemical death!" Eagles are back in the news, desperately warning us about the lead infiltrating and poisoning their warrior bodies. As we failed to listen in the 1960s, I fear we will fail to listen now.

On February 26, 1975, my husband and I finally called it quits, and he left me with the children. In March, I forged ahead with my longtime dream to purchase ten acres in the West Virginia countryside. It was time for a change, but I had no idea how difficult it would be as a divorcée with three young children.

Our home was built in the center of what had been a cornfield, and our water source was a shallow well that drained into the farmer's pond. Michael was five years old, Sarah was three, and I was about five months pregnant with Clint.

The children and I enjoyed living in the country, despite its being physically demanding for me. Michael and Sarah were overjoyed to finally have a dog, which our cramped apartment living had denied them. We adopted a gentle, intelligent border collie named Sparks from the humane society.

Sparks did not add to my workload, as Michael did a surprisingly good job of caring for him. Looking back, I marvel at how mature Michael was, not just in caring for Sparks but in looking out for his sister and helping me in countless ways.

But without my husband, country life was far more demanding than I had anticipated. To my consternation, I learned that even with a garden tractor, mowing required about an hour per acre per week, three seasons of the year. In winter, shoveling snow sufficiently to get my car in and out of the driveway exhausted me some days. I had underestimated the amount of time required to drive back into town to drop off the children with our longtime babysitter, Mrs. Claiborne, so I could continue to work.

I was an accounting assistant for Campbell and Klein, the father-and-daughter law firm where I had been employed while my husband completed his bachelor's degree in computer science at Liberty College. The plan had been for me to stay at home with the children and pursue my own bachelor's degree in journalism through an online course. Oh, well. Things rarely go as people plan.

Overall, I was glad enough to have many activities to keep me occupied. I had my hands full, keeping the well, the car, and our tight budget functioning, all while keeping the children clean, fed, clothed, entertained, and taxied to and from Mrs. Claiborne's.

I do not know that I've ever grieved the loss of my marriage as I should have done. He was a highly intelligent man and a good husband and father, but his plans didn't turn out as he'd hoped either.

I kept up a crazy pace through my pregnancy and Clint's delivery. By the time we celebrated Clint's first birthday, I'd nearly collapsed from exhaustion and had to list the property for sale.

When Clint was eighteen months old, we moved back to Charleston.

With his dark curly hair and intense blue eyes, Clint was an adorable baby. He quickly grew into a happy toddler: active, energetic, and busy. Maybe I should have recognized signs of issues. In stark contrast with his siblings, who delighted in the stories I enjoyed penning for them to supplement standard children's literature, little Clint hated to have anyone read anything to him.

"Stop it, Mommy!" he would say, as if my efforts were a torture for him.

Now that we were back in town and I had more time with the children, I increasingly noticed Clint's difficulty functioning in situations with background noise, and although I didn't think much of the fact that he often completely ignored Sarah's calling to him to come see a robin out the window or Michael's asking him to play a game, I did start noticing that he didn't seem to hear when I asked him to do simple things.

"Hand Mommy the towel, Clint. Clint, honey, hand Mommy the wet towel, please," I requested. I was cleaning the bathroom sink and reached out, expecting him to respond.

But Clint continued sliding the rubber ducky along the edge of the tub, as if I hadn't even spoken.

When Clint turned four, I enrolled him in a Montessori preschool.

After a few months, Clint's teacher, Mrs. Bell, called me in for a conference.

After we had shaken hands and introduced ourselves, I squeezed into the small desk across from her imposing one and waited expectantly.

Mrs. Bell looked down at some notes on a legal pad and then back up at me a moment before speaking. "Mrs. Marshall, I don't know exactly how to tell you this ..."

"Just tell me," I suggested, carefully keeping my tone neutral and nondefensive.

"Mrs. Marshall," she began again, "I suspect that Clint has some learning disabilities. Clint struggles to learn, which makes him difficult in the classroom."

Although her mentioning Clint's learning challenges was not entirely unexpected, I could barely refrain from protesting that Mrs. Bell had labeled my sweet boy as difficult!

I was polite, but my heart hurt for my precious son.

Life was good in our suburban house. Michael and Sarah made friends readily in the neighborhood, consistently brought home good grades, and continued to meet or exceed all of my expectations. I praised them, of course, but perhaps not as enthusiastically as I would have done if Clint hadn't always been watching me closely, reading my lips, and trailing a few steps behind his siblings.

Clint was a free spirit. He made friends with everyone. He was always smiling and busy. Adults and teachers didn't always appreciate his happy-go-lucky attitude. Over time, they destroyed his trust. Within a few short months of starting school, he no longer made eye contact with them.

When Clint entered kindergarten, I asked the school district to begin testing for learning disabilities.

"We recommend that testing wait until he gets into grade school," Mrs. Proctor said firmly, closing the conversation almost as soon as it had begun.

I put up a weak argument, really more of a plea, as Mrs. Proctor led me to the door of her office and showed me out.

As a good mom who did not want to rock the boat unduly by challenging professionals' authority, I did not pursue this avenue further.

However, during the three-year wait for educational professionals to test my son, I arranged for testing at the Charleston Area Medical Center (CAMC) Women and Children's Hospital.

CAMC identified five learning disabilities, none of which amounted to much of anything when considered on their individual merits. Taken together, however, five seemed to be quite overwhelming and constituted what the hospital warned could mean "serious trouble." Clint's main challenge was labeled *auditory processing disorder* (or *central auditory processing disorder*).

People afflicted with this disorder do not recognize subtle differences between sounds in words. They find it difficult to stay focused on verbal or auditory stimuli and may process thoughts or ideas slowly and have difficulty articulating what they think. Figurative language tends to confuse them.

A hospital doctor explained, "Imagine you are standing down inside a well. It's a little hollow with the sounds echoing off the walls. Someone drops a couple of pebbles. Someone says 'Hellooo.' This would not bother a normal person. But for Clint, it causes great discomfort. Clint has frayed auditory nerve endings."

Before I had time to react to this, he added, "Furthermore, nothing can be done; it's permanent. He will never learn to read any better than an eighth grader. The other issues will make it almost impossible for him to learn in a classroom setting."

Reeling at this news, I found the doctor's shrug surreal.

Clint could hear, but he could not hear distinct word sounds. It was as if white noise was too loud for him to distinguish the difference between "then" and "when." Instead, he read lips. He could not hear the differences in vowel sounds, and sometimes he could not hear consonants at all.

If a speaker's back was to Clint, he could not understand what was said. Therefore, when a teacher was writing on the blackboard, Clint did not hear the instructions. He was always in trouble for "not listening."

Childhood developmental tests explained many things, including why he hated being read bedtime stories.

The school granted Clint access to the special resource room at school but otherwise did not help in any meaningful way. I hired the learning disability (LD) teacher to tutor him two days a week before school and a second teacher to tutor him after school for two days a week to cover his classroom lessons.

Meanwhile, Michael graduated high school at seventeen and launched into his life with enthusiasm. Having earned a scholarship, he went to MIT in Cambridge and never again lived at home. He met Paula Warren when they were both freshmen. They dated all through college and married shortly after their graduation from the five-year engineering program. Together, they began building their careers and, shortly thereafter, a family of their own.

Sarah had just turned eighteen when she graduated from high school. Uninterested in the scholarship offer she received, my daughter continued living at home while she spent a year working at the Clay Center for the Arts and Sciences, considering her options. She eventually chose an undergraduate program at the University of California and moved to the West Coast. After graduating with a bachelor's degree in criminal justice, she started her first professional job as a research assistant in a law office, where she met attorney Mark Stone, whom she later married. Eventually, they moved to Florida.

Clint worked hard to learn and graduated high school when he was nineteen. Tall and handsome with his dark curly hair and bright blue eyes, he was the picture of health, and I was very proud of him.

His off-and-on girlfriend, Tara Waggoner, often joined us for dinner. Clint helped her keep her old VW running, and she helped him bury Sparks in the backyard when our longtime companion passed away.

The CAMC tests had shown that Clint possessed remarkable mechanical ability, which, the doctor had predicted, "should make it reasonably easy for him to earn a living." Perhaps in 1981, that had been the case. But by 1997, things had changed.

Clint found it difficult to fill out job applications. It was also becoming increasingly difficult to get a manual labor job without a college degree. Clint simply couldn't go to college. The local vocational school (where Tara was studying accounting) wouldn't accept him, saying he was too advanced for any special vocational training in his areas of interest. He was one of those kids to whom society refers as having fallen through the cracks.

two

A Promising Future

While continuing to live at home, Clint struggled to find a place to work and be happy.

I told him, "Take a job and learn everything you can. When you have finished learning, quit and get a new job. Learn everything you can at that new job, and when you have learned it all, quit and get another new job."

Working various construction and maintenance jobs was his college.

One of his high school friends unkindly remarked, "What's wrong with you that you can't keep a job, Clint? Gee! You're such a loser."

I told Clint, "Until someone walks in your boots, they'll never have anything positive to say."

Clint did what he had to do. Marshaling his excellent mechanical abilities, he became a highly qualified pipe fitter. By the time he was twenty-nine years old, he was earning a nice living, traveling around the United States from job to job.

He had a red Chevy truck with heavy-duty suspension that allowed him to load up all of his tools and his motor dirt bike, camping gear, and fishing equipment and ease on down the road.

By then, companies were calling him regularly, and he had a couple of traveling friends. They found work while also finding time to play.

I finally felt confident that Clint's future was bright.

tHREE

What Really Happened

Did Clint fall in to manual labor because he could not read well? Was it because companies intentionally used him? I have no idea. But I firmly believe Clint was exposed to dangerous caustic chemicals without his knowledge. "How do you know this?" you may ask.

I can say for a fact that directly after an unknown liquid poured out of a pipe that he was told to cut, Clint became deathly ill for days. This happened not once but several times, and coincidence only stretches so far. Pipe demolition was a large part of his job.

The pipes were supposed to have been back-flushed to remove any dangerous chemicals. College-degreed safety engineers are trained to make sure of that, but apparently, they are not always successful. I know now that mistakes like this are covered up—and companies send exposed workers home. After a few days of illness, they return to work.

Until his job working at Ultra, Clint was never sent back to a facility that caused an exposure. He was never told the truth about the materials to which he had been exposed. If he asked too many questions, he was asked, "Do you want to keep your job? Decide what is more important. That spill happened last week. It's over; you're okay."

I wish I had known then what I know now. Such exposures are residual and cause major liver damage. (Essentially, those exposures are the reason for this book.)

Clint worked at chemical plants, as well as at plants that produced silicon wafers. He worked for steel distributors and auto parts manufacturers. In fact, he worked at no fewer than a dozen plants where he risked being exposed to deadly chemicals.

Clint and I believe we know exactly when his TILT (toxicant-induced loss of tolerance) began. At one particular plant, no one told him to what he was being exposed. No one gave him a respirator or protective clothing. Never was a safety engineer on duty to protect him. While safety engineers are employees of the company and charged with protecting the workers, they first protect the companies that pay their salaries.

fOUR

The First Symptoms (2003–2004)

In 2003, Clint was twenty-seven years old. He had learned the construction world the hard way—through much work.

He was hired to work as part of a subcontracted crew as a maintenance man at the ULTRA plant in Pennsylvania. ULTRA manufactures electronic-grade silicon wafers for the semiconductor industry. Their wafers are used by companies all over the world to make integrated circuits and semiconductor devices that power a myriad electronic products, from computers to cell phones to digital watches and automobile engine systems.

Not long after Clint began working at ULTRA, the plant superintendent discovered that Clint was more than a maintenance person. Recognizing Clint's high mechanical ability, the supervisor made Clint the go-to guy.

ULTRA was moving their entire Washington State plant to Pennsylvania. They had to ship large water-cleaning machines across the United States on flatbed semis. Some machines were used to remove arsenic and other toxic waste from the water, created during the doping process. Other machines made the wafers.

Doping is how manufacturers create semiconductors. It involves adding an impurity (e.g., barium) to a pure chemical (usually silicon) to create an imbalance in the electronic fields. This creates semiconductors.

When Clint first contacted ULTRA about his increasing ill health in 2011, rather than helping him get the medical answers he desperately needed, they chose to respond as adversaries and turned him away. Therefore, I am forced to base my findings on assumptions rather than facts that ULTRA should have shared immediately. I welcome ULTRA to compensate Clint for that damage at any time, but all these years later, we still wait.

My research revealed that ULTRA had been asked to leave Washington State. Indeed, their plant eventually became a Superfund cleanup site. On the internet, I found the company's alarming polluting scorecard and other damning reports. The company had been cited for releasing hydrochloric acid, one of the most hazardous compounds (i.e., among the worst 10 percent) to our ecosystem and human health.

For the following important reasons, I want to share, in greater depth, Clint's working situation with ULTRA:

> Several of his coworkers (and friends) who worked there are now dead.
>
> Clint worked longer at that location than any other so far in his career. Strange things went on while he was working there.
>
> He was hired by a company to work in maintenance, but his employer did not instruct him on what to do. ULTRA's plant superintendent told him to do work that was above and beyond plant

maintenance.

Because of the layering of supervision, no one accepts responsibility for Clint's condition or for that of any other construction person who worked there.

One man has been suffering a slow and miserable death since 2007 (as a doctor predicted in 2011 for Clint's future). He refuses to hear the truth (though we have not given up trying to share with his family what we have learned).

Clint started working at ULTRA in November 2003. He was in perfect health, never missed a day of work, and was never sick.

As Clint pulled through the company's front gate, he saw a perfectly designed building. In front of the building, geese and ducks inhabited a peaceful lake. Everything seemed picture-perfect at first glance: a beautiful, modern building and an impeccably manicured lawn. The entire plant was surrounded by a high security fence. A security guard checked the credentials of anyone entering through the front gate before granting access to the property. The guard used a mirror to inspect underneath everyone's vehicle.

Clint initially felt like he must have made a wrong turn. He couldn't be in the right place with that much high security. Clint was in the right place for his job—and in the wrong place for his life.

As time went on, the job crew expanded, as men from other companies arrived. He recognized some of them from past job sites and remarked that it often felt like a workers' reunion.

For the first few weeks, Clint took orders from his official employer, Century Construction, which had brought in his crew to perform maintenance. The longer he worked there, however, the more he was instructed by the ULTRA maintenance supervisor, rather than Century.

Clint did his job very well and soon was working in the clean rooms that manufactured computer chips by utilizing a doping process. As previously mentioned, doping involves adding an impurity, such as barium, to a pure chemical, usually silicon, to create an imbalance in the electronic fields. The process is repeated many times. Eventually, this creates semiconductors.

Clint noticed a temporary work-to-hire janitor who spent his days walking along the property. Clint called this man "the Russian."

After conversing with the Russian, Clint discovered that the man had a US visa work permit. The Russian spent his time gathering birds that had died, having flown through plumes of white steam that came out of the roofing vents—the same roofing vents that Clint's coworkers had recently installed.

Clint wondered, *Why would ULTRA hire a person who could barely speak English and was from a temporary employment company to pick up dead birds?*

Clint often noticed flocks of blackbirds flying above the plant. As these birds flew over the exhaust vents, he would observe fifteen or more of the birds at a time plummet from the sky, literally dropping dead. What chemicals were being exhausted that were deadly enough to kill the birds within a few seconds?

Clint asked the foreman, "What's going on with all these birds dying?"

The foreman told him sternly, "That is none of your concern. Just do the job you're being paid to do, or go home."

Since Clint was a contracted disposable employee who desperately needed his job, he stayed quiet and kept working.

Over time, Clint noticed that some of the men who were working on the roof were getting sick and going home. Some didn't come back.

Every day there was a hose that ran out the emergency door. Unless an inspection was scheduled, the doors were always propped open. He figured out that this was necessary in order to flush out the system. When the water-cleaning machines were scrubbed, the chemicals and wastewater were put into a transport vehicle and taken to an environmental dump site. Any remaining fluids were flushed out through the hose onto the blacktop, which then ran down into the river below. Men moved the hose and reattached it as each machine was maintained.

One day, while the Russian was scooping dead fish from the lake in front of the building, Clint talked to him about the dead fish and birds.

The Russian said, "This is nothing! This plant killed *everything* in the lake a short time ago. The lake had to be drained."

More special trade workers began to show up to work on the machines that were being brought in for the expansion. One day, an electrician cut through a piece of conduit, and the power was shut off to parts of the building. The backup generator that was part of the expansion for emergency situations was not in working condition. I wondered, *How did this company get a permit with these potential dangers and no emergency systems in place?*

As a result of the power loss, the rooms were evacuated immediately. The building was filling up with the exhaust that should have been venting through the roof—the same exhaust that kills birds.

During routine maintenance, Clint specifically recalls sticking his hand into a machine—and pulling out crushed wafer-like objects. The supervisor told Clint to remove the broken chips in order to free a clog. Unfortunately, this machine cleaned arsenic, barium, and other toxins from water. No gloves or safety gear were recommended or provided. Clint was never told with what he was coming in contact.

Winter 2003

Repair and demolition of the existing exhaust vents was part of the maintenance contract ULTRA had with Century Construction.

When Clint removed the first piece of the duct and threw it to the ground, the plant supervisor rushed over, shouting, "Don't throw that stuff down! Be careful. It has exhaust residue in it." As he continued the work, more and more dust particles went down the inside of Clint's shirt. He specifically recalls cutting the pipe and watching as dirty sediment became airborne and settled on the ceiling tile below.

Clint's skin burned as the dust particles landed on him. He immediately called for the supervisor, who directed Clint and the other workers to get down from the exhaust vents. He took Clint to the maintenance room to examine his skin.

"That's not so bad. Go home, Clint. Take the rest of the day off. You'll be fine tomorrow," the supervisor assured him. I believe this person knew what chemical had burned Clint's skin.

My question is, why weren't the workers given protective, hazmat suits? The time off was taken without pay. This is the norm in the construction world, yet we may wonder why fewer people are choosing skilled trades as their career choices.

Spring 2004

When the supervisor had given him his work order, Clint took the stairs to the second floor and walked to the mechanical room. He needed to climb a ladder, remove a ceiling panel, and climb into the access area. He crawled to the ceiling area above an office, where two women were working. His job was to follow some vent pipes that hung over the clean-room area and find a clog. The section was dark; he had to use a flashlight. After finding the vent pipes that came from the first-floor clean rooms, he had to cut the pipes in different places, hoping to find the clog.

While he was cutting into the pipe, dirty sediment again became airborne. He watched the as the particles fell onto the women working below. He remembered the incident from October 2003, when the same particles went down his shirt and burned his back.

He stared down through the ceiling, watching the two ladies sitting at their desks below. They had no idea that they just had been exposed to dangerous toxins.

To this day, Clint feels horrible about what he saw happen. There is a good possibility that those women are now very ill.

fIVE

Pipe Fitting

While working in the same location, Clint was standing on a ten-foot ladder, demolishing a pipe, when he came in contact with a solution of hydrogen fluoride in water. The pipe had not been drained as the supervisor had assured him it had.

While Clint was cutting the pipe, the red Sawzall (a reciprocating saw) started to turn pink, and the black handle began changing to a grayish white.

Seeing Clint throw down the Sawzall, the supervisor came running. He rushed Clint to the restroom and gave him some unidentified product to put on his skin. Again, Clint was sent home for a couple of days to recuperate—again, without pay.

When he returned to the same job and asked if the fluid had been hydrofluoric acid, the foreman frowned and gave a small nod. "You'll have to keep quiet or go home," he said. "Everything's under control."

six

Unloading and Setting Up Large Machinery

Clint was often asked to go to the delivery area to look at a piece of equipment that had been delivered on a flatbed truck. ULTRA asked Clint which tools were needed to get the machine up and working. Again, time was money when it came to the machines operating. Clint was in charge of scoping the work and making sure the required parts were available, so the equipment could be piped in quickly. However, this was not what Century hired him to do. He was hired for building maintenance, not skilled pipe fitting. ULTRA, not Century, was directing his work. In my view, this makes ULTRA responsible for Clint's knocking on heaven's door.

As he and three other men transported the machine, Clint noticed that it was full of the same white residue that had burned his back months earlier.

As he worked, Clint saw increasing evidence that most of the equipment had been used previously.

"Is this load from another plant?" Clint asked the semi-truck driver.

"Yeah," the driver confirmed.

"Where?"

"Washington State," the driver replied before returning his attention to paperwork on a clipboard.

Clint did as he was told. He had no other choice, unless he wanted to quit. Then what? Find another job with another big-dollar company that would do the same? After all, this was how it had been from the first job Clint ever accepted. He was disposable. People hired to protect the disposable employees earned their salary by protecting the large corporation, not the hourly paid laborers that society thinks they protect.

Seven

Covering Up the Scrubber Explosion (2004–2005)

Rumor was that the machine that cleaned the arsenic out of the water had blown up the previous night. Toxic water had spewed all over the floor, sprayed the ceiling, and run down the walls. The machine operator had shut it down and brought in a hose through a set of doors to start draining. ULTRA management controlled the cleanup and did not report anything about it to the EPA.

On this ominous day, Clint walked to the back of the building and noticed water on the ground, and the emergency doors were both propped open. The Russian and a few others were sweeping out the water.

Later that morning, ULTRA's main plant supervisor came to the Century Construction job trailer and asked if Clint thought he could repair the clean-water machine.

He took Clint to the machine that had blown up the previous night. For some time, Clint tried to braze (solder) the split and cracked copper tubes. Then he went to the break room.

"The brazing rods don't seem to be working," he told ULTRA's maintenance man.

"Keep trying," the man replied.

While Clint was doing just that, the supervisor tapped on the door and handed Clint different rods. Clint thought that was a little strange—that all the engineers would not enter the room where he was working. The supervisor only tapped on the door, opened it, handed Clint the new rods, quickly said "Use these," and shut the door—all in a matter of seconds.

During his next break, ULTRA engineers invaded the trailer. They were adamant that the machine could not stay shut down. They rattled off how much money per hour it was costing while the machine was not in production.

Clint worked the rest of the day with no break. He fixed the leaks, and the toxic water was flowing again.

Clint spent over eight hours working in that machine, despite the NIOSH (National Institute for Occupational Safety and Health) rules on how long a person can stay in an area without a clean air supply. The time limits are minutes, not hours. OSHA (Occupational Safety and Health Administration) specifies that there should be a break of a certain number of hours between exposures and requires workers to wear chemical-hazard protective clothing. Because ULTRA refuses to talk to us, we have no idea to what Clint actually was exposed. Therefore, we will never know which NIOSH rules pertain to this situation.

The machine was made of copper. Arsenic- or maybe barium-poisoned water ran through that machine until the water was clean enough to be recycled.

This had been a very dangerous job. Although Clint did not know this at the time, we can assume the engineers did know because they limited their own exposure time.

Clint was not given any protective gear. He wore nothing but his usual work clothes. The company engineers explained what the problems were and what needed to be done but never came into the room while Clint was working. Because ULTRA oversaw this entire process, they are directly responsible for Clint's (then near future) health issues. In the absence of willing witnesses, Clint has found it impossible to prove it even happened.

When he was finished, they tested the machine, and everyone was surprised at what he had been able to do. It took Clint years to realize it was not admiration for his skill level but because they knew he would soon be very sick.

Note: The hobbyist and nonprofessional welder is strongly warned with regard to rods and flux (the material that coats the welding rods.) Many different trades beyond just welders are potentially affected by heavy-metal toxicity and poisoning. Those involved in plumbing, iron working, and pipe fitting also are affected, but the warnings are assumed to be known in the trades.

Eight

Other Incidents

Clint noticed many strange occurrences while working at the plant. For example, names of men who had been injured would disappear from the sign-in sheets. Clint recalled working with one of those men (number nine on the security check-in list) while fabricating a pipe. He worked with him for an entire day. The following day, number nine worked with another pipe fitter. Clint met them for lunch. At the end of the day, Clint heard that number nine had gotten extremely sick while working on the roof vents. Clint had just been on that roof, where the vents spewed something that killed birds.

"Where did number nine go?" Clint asked the next day.

"He worked for a temp placement agency. I don't know where he is," a ULTRA foreman told him dismissively.

This man had gotten deathly ill, coughing and gagging. His face turning a putrid shade of yellow. Three weeks later, another welder from the same temp agency told Clint that number nine had been diagnosed with serious kidney problems.

Clint described the roof vents as an interesting blend of different shapes and sizes, with exhaust vents at odd angles. Now Clint suspects that the company may have done this in an attempt to escape EPA clean-air-quality detection.

Clint has told me quite a bit about the use of hydrofluoric acid, a very strong inorganic acid used for industrial purposes for metal cleaning, etching, and electronics manufacturing. This kind of acid eats the skin, causing severe burns. It also destroys calcium in the body. It is an acute poison that can cause immediate and permanent damage to the lungs and corneas of the eyes. In its concentrated form, it interferes with calcium metabolism. It may also cause systemic toxicity and eventual cardiac arrest. It can be fatal—with a dosage of as little as 160 cm^2, which covers twenty-five square inches of skin.

After news got out that Clint was able to braze the water machine, he was offered a job with one of the companies that had a crew working at ULTRA. Clint took the job and moved to a new job site in July 2004.

July 2004

At the end of another workday, I was in the kitchen preparing dinner when I heard the garage door go up. "Hi, Clint! How was your day?" I called.

"Wow!" he hollered up the basement stairs as he prepared to take a shower. "What a great day! Remember when I repaired that water machine? Well, based on that success, someone just offered me a real pipe-fitting job. Did you hear me? A real pipe-fitting job! I told you no one thought I could do it. I did it, and I just got a real job. I'm taking a shower. What's for dinner? I'm starved. What a great day!"

Clint came up from his shower and enjoyed our simple dinner of baked chicken, scalloped potatoes, and tossed salad. "And I'll be getting two dollars more an hour. Yahoo!"

Clint cleaned up the dinner dishes, and I went into my office to log onto my employer's site to review that day's work.

By this time, Garin Winston had become more than a good friend to me. Garin, a self-employed project management consultant, had come into my life when he oversaw a major upgrade to Campbell and Klein's computer systems and procedures. He was smart, polite, and often made me laugh. We enjoyed verbal sparring and had many interests—such as camping, cooking, and astronomy—in common. In short order, Garin became someone I talked to daily and someone with whom I could discuss everything, from investments to celestial events. Eventually, he convinced me to try freelancing too, on my own schedule and according to clients' needs.

Although Campbell and Klein remained my clients, I began working with many small companies as an accounting software consultant. In less than a year's time, my work had evolved into freelance copywriting, editing, and website development. By and large, if my clients had work, I had work. I was able to work out at the gym three times a week and to go camping or on weekend getaways with Garin. I was working fewer hours and realizing more income.

Life was good.

"Mom, I'm going out to cut the grass," Clint yelled as the garage door went back down.

August 2004

At the end of another workday, I heard the garage door go up. Today was for celebration; Sarah and Mark had made me a grandma.

"Hi, Clint! How was your day?"

"Just great!" he said as he headed into the shower.

"Garin and I are leaving for Florida today to go see my grandbaby. Not sure when I'll be home. I'm just about ready to go."

"While you're gone, I think I will demo this basement. It is going to be a messy job, so it'll be better if no one is home. I want to pull off this old paneling and rip out the carpet. I want to paint the walls and the floor. Is that okay with you?"

"Sure! Knock yourself out. Oh, and Clint—there's a pot of spaghetti on the stove. Please remember to store any leftovers. Okay, I'm out of here. Have fun with your remodeling," I headed out the door with my suitcase. I planned to pick up Garin on my way to the airport.

During that trip, Garin suggested marriage, and I told him I would think about it. He was a good, solid, caring companion, reliable and kind. Our relationship worked well. We encouraged and supported one another. Yes, I would think about it.

Ten days later, when I came home with many precious photos and my heart full of happy memories and plans, I was dismayed to find that things had not gone well in my absence.

During his demo, Clint had tripped over an extension cord and run his hand into a fan. His fingers had had to be pinned and sewn back on.

At work, he was assigned to the shop for time to recover.

My life was busy with work, the gym, and friends. I did not especially take note when Clint began to feel unwell.

Later, he confessed his stomach was chronically upset, and he felt like he had a touch of the flu. His skin tingled and seemed to him to be subtly changing in color. He had itchy skin rashes that burned. He blamed it all on the hand trauma and didn't tell me any of this at the time.

Clint went back to work in the field as a pipe fitter by the middle of September.

October 2004

The garage door went up, signaling the end of another workday.

"Mom, I'm home," Clint called as he headed for the shower. "I leave in a few days for San Diego to work at the Coors plant. Go figure! Me, getting to go to San Diego to work! They're going to fly me out there, and I get to stay in a hotel! The work will be really easy. I'll be installing poly tubing that controls air actuators for conveyor belts. My company is sending me there to give my hand more time to heal. This is really sweet!"

In the days that followed, as he continued to work, Clint became sicker. His sensation of having stomach flu grew, rather than diminished. He had night sweats. The rash spread and made him feel like his skin was on fire; still, he told me nothing about it.

January 2005

"Mom, I'm home," Clint called, heading for the shower. "I leave in a few days for the ravioli plant in Louisiana. It's going to be another easy job. No heavy lifting and no chemicals. I haven't been feeling very well lately, so it's good that I'm getting a break from dirty work environments."

I was surprised to hear him say he wasn't feeling well. Clint never got sick. He was a powerful machine.

"What's going on?" I asked. My right hand held a noodle, suspended above the baking dish, where I was preparing lasagna.

He brushed it off as no big deal. "I'm sure it will go away, Mom. I don't feel right, but it's hard to explain."

I later discovered he was not being honest. He was throwing up every morning and having night sweats that included chills and fever. He just didn't want me to worry. Mostly, I didn't.

March 2005

"I'm home," Clint called, as he always did. "Tomorrow I move to a Tyson food processing plant. I'll be replacing screw pipe for steam coils. I love this job. Since I left ULTRA, I haven't come in contact with any chemicals. It's been all food plants." He sounded genuinely happy about this, but then his tone changed. "I just don't understand why I can't feel better."

"Have you gone to the doctor?" I asked.

"No. I don't know how to explain how I feel. It comes and goes. Sometimes I feel like I have the flu. Other days aren't bad, and every once in a while, I even feel all right. It's just too hard to explain. I know it sounds crazy."

April 2005

Garin convinced me to take a vacation with him to Hawaii. That was the most beautiful and most romantic week of my life. We went sailing, snorkeling, and hiking. We toured Pearl Harbor and the dormant volcano at Diamond Head crater.

One lovely evening, while dancing at a nightclub in Honolulu, Garin caught me with my defenses down. I agreed we could plan to be married in May 2006.

A few minutes later, when we had stepped out onto the balcony, Garin surprised me by getting down on one knee and slipping a beautiful ring on my finger.

"You've made me the happiest man in the world, Peggy," he said gruffly.

"Get up, Garin!" I said with a laugh.

We discussed Garin's selling his condo and moving in with Clint and me. The house was spacious enough for Garin to use a spare bedroom for his home office. We discussed wedding reception venues and guest lists. I felt like all was right with the world.

In fact, for some weeks after my fiancé and I returned to the mainland, I continued making wedding plans, blissfully unaware of the time bomb ticking under my own roof.

May 2005

"Mom, I'm home," Clint said. "I'm going to Parkersburg next. This is new construction—some prefabricated pipe installation, some metal stairs, and bolt-up work. It will be a good mix of things to do. I'm going to take my bike and camping gear. I think I'll feel better if I stay outside, work and play."

"You're still not feeling any better?" I asked, turning down the heat on the salmon patties to quiet the sound of sizzling for a moment.

"No, not really," he said. "I just can't seem to shake whatever this is."

Clint camped some of the time and spent some nights at the hotel. Working in extreme heat was taking its toll. Clint later told me he was having diarrhea and throwing up more and more. If he missed work and stayed in the hotel air conditioning, he would feel a little better and would go back to work—only to feel sick again.

He even began to look sick, and his foreman told him to see a doctor. Finally, Clint went to the urgent care medical center in Parkersburg. The doctor there told him to go home. Something unspecified was "really wrong." Unwilling to voice his suspicions, the doctor just said Clint's condition was outside his scope of ability to treat. Clint came home and went to his doctor.

Dr. Hanes diagnosed a urinary tract infection and prescribed antibiotics. A technician drew Clint's blood.

Test results showed raised levels of bilirubin, an orange-yellow pigment formed in the liver by the breakdown of hemoglobin and excreted in bile. The doctor diagnosed "symptoms involving skin and other integumentary tissue, jaundice, unspecified, not of newborn." Clint's blood also showed that he had elevated levels of arsenic. The doctor had no explanation whatsoever for the rash and planned to test Clint again in a week.

I heard the garage door go up. "Mom, I'm sick," Clint called from the basement as he headed to the shower.

"What are you doing home? Is the job over? Is something wrong?" I asked with a wrench of pain in my own stomach.

Clint came upstairs for dinner. His skin looked yellow, except for large brown circles beneath his sunken eyes. He said it felt like he had to urinate all the time, but he could not. He couldn't keep down any food and hadn't been able to sleep.

"Mom, I feel like crap. Doc Hanes says I have a bladder and kidney infection, and I will be better in a few days. I'll go back to Parkersburg on Sunday." He seemed defeated. "I still don't know what's causing this rash."

"What happened?" I asked him, worried.

"Remember when I said I just wasn't feeling well? It just won't go away. Ever since I worked on that tank at ULTRA, I just keep feeling sick. It's like something has crawled inside of me, and it's killing me slowly. I don't understand the bladder infection. Isn't that what girls get?" he said, obviously upset. "I made a terrible mistake a few nights ago. I stayed at a campground and woke up, sick, in the middle of the night. I had run out of water. I went to the campground water fountain. The next morning, I saw a "Not Potable" sign on that fountain. What does that mean? Do you think that made me sick?"

Fighting down panic, I told myself it would be okay. Clint was strong. He would be okay; he just needed rest. I served him dinner and sent him to bed. That night, neither of us slept.

Late Sunday night, Clint drove back to work. He was still sick.

When the phone rang, I answered, half expecting it to be Clint, telling me he was unwell. But it was Garin, delighted to report that he had sold the condo. It seemed like a million years ago since he and I had decided that he would sell his condo and move in with Clint and me. I'm not sure what I actually said, but I remember thinking, *That's just great, honey. I don't have time to deal with it, though.*

Two weeks later, Clint was home sick, just like before. Antibiotics worked as long as the prescription lasted; then the urinary infection symptoms returned. Even the doctor was confused. Clint didn't test positive for an infection, but he still tested with high levels of bilirubin and arsenic. The doctor ordered another round of tests.

Between doctor visits, Clint returned to work in Parkersburg.

When the next set of test results came back, the doctor called Clint and told him to come home immediately. Clint had tested positive for another urinary tract infection. His doctor gave up and referred him to a urologist.

This was the first of many doctors who refused to listen. Clint kept asking him about the high levels of arsenic and bilirubin reported on his previous tests. His doctor refused to comment on those results. Why?

June 2005

Garin moved in, and we compromised on combining all of our belongings. We gave away my old dishes in favor of using his, and we sold his sectional sofa since I already had two comfortable sofas in the den. Garin tacked down a plywood floor in the attic to provide storage for the rest of our surplus belongings. We started making plans for our wedding as a normal couple, living normal lives.

In reality, I rode a mad carousel for years. For a few measures, Garin and I rode elegant chargers, side by side, holding hands in the sunlight.

We attended a Yanni concert and took an overnight trip to Lake Hope in McArthur, Ohio. Then Clint and I clung to one another in terror as the merry-go-round spun counterclockwise through a house of horrors. Doctors and nurses approached with the appearance of angels, only to turn into demons as they reached out for us. No! The demons did not reach out for us but for Clint, only for Clint! I felt like I was the only thing standing between my son and his utter annihilation.

In between these extremes, I worked for an increasing number of clients and tried to remain calm. I rejoiced when Garin and Clint were able to pass the potatoes like family, and I reacted angrily when they yelled over who forgot to return a screwdriver to the junk drawer.

September 2005

I heard the garage door go up. "Mom, I'm home," Clint called from the basement as he headed for the shower. "Because I've been so sick, I've been moved into the shop. I'll be making deliveries. My testicles hurt, and my back is killing me. I have my first appointment with the urologist tomorrow. I sure hope he can figure this out."

My chest felt tight. Something was seriously wrong. I began to wonder if his symptoms could be caused by heavy-metal poisoning. I counseled myself against overreacting. *Calm down. You will figure this out. Think, think, think!*

His pain and symptoms continued to intensify. He stayed in the shop for six weeks.

It had been a year since he first began to feel sick, a year since we started on this mystery journey. His blood tests were still showing "elevated bilirubin with symptoms involving skin and other integumentary tissue, jaundice, unspecified, not of newborn."

Why were doctors ignoring that? Clint was more ill every day, and something was very wrong.

I began to search on the internet for heavy-metal poisoning. I found an article titled "Welding Fume Lawsuits" by Brayton Purcell in October 2003. "An Illinois jury awarded Lawrence Elam, a 65-year-old man with Parkinson's disease, $1 million based on his exposure to manganese-containing welding fumes. Three welding rod companies were named in his lawsuit ..."

By 2015, Clint's urgent need for medical answers was ending. Sadly, on June 2015 the following was released on the internet:

> The steering committees for the parties in the Welding Fume MDL have reached a global settlement resolving nearly all welding fume cases pending in state or federal courts. The settlement is a substantial victory for the welding industry and will practically end welding fume litigation as a mass tort.
>
> In exchange for dismissing their lawsuits and releasing all manufacturers, distributors, and sellers of welding fume products from liability, the participating plaintiffs will be eligible to receive payments from a settlement pool being funded by welding rod manufacturers. Nearly all plaintiffs have opted to participate, and the settlement will result in the dismissal of nearly 95 percent of all currently pending welding fume cases. A handful of plaintiffs elected to proceed with their lawsuits, which are expected to go to trial within the next 12 months.
>
> The settlement will result in the dismissal and release of distributors of welding products, even though the settlement is being funded entirely by the manufacturers. This will not prevent the filing of new cases by other

welders in the future. However, it is anticipated that the difficult track record experienced by welding fume plaintiffs over the last nine years will be a significant disincentive for future mass tort litigation, especially for welders with questionable claims. The settlement essentially concludes welding fume litigation as a mass tort, which began in 2003. At its peak, nearly 14,000 welding fume exposure claims were pending in state and federal courts. By 2005, welding fume litigation was being touted as the "next asbestos." The industry fought back and was vindicated. Since 2003, the industry won more than thirty trials, while losing just five. Of the five jury verdicts awarded to plaintiffs, only one survived appeal. (http://www.weldingandgasestoday.org)

If you read only one part of this book, read this:

It has become apparent that many people have suffered from everyday low-dose exposure to environmental toxicants and chemicals. The TILT theory, first identified by Dr. Claudia S. Miller, states that some of the environmental exposures can even affect genes and DNA. Once a gene has been exposed, it is difficult to turn off that sensitivity.

There are multiple episodes of environmental contamination, and those are the ones that the public is aware of. There are most likely many more contaminants that the public is unaware of. Clint and I are desperately trying to get help and exposure for those who suffer currently—and for those who are unable to find the answers they need.

According to an article in the November 2013 issue of *Discovery* magazine, Gulf War veterans suffer from TILT as well. According to this article, their illnesses were the subject of long-term controversy. The military wants us to believe in PTSD—posttraumatic stress disorder—

rather than neurotoxicity. Neurotoxicity is the damage that occurs to the brain and the peripheral nervous system from toxic chemicals. Symptoms for brain toxicity include things like:

Short-term memory loss
Loss of circulation
Body out of Balances
Flu-like symptoms

Clint's symptoms align with those symptoms. He had a flu that never went away, and the soft tissue pain nearly destroyed his pelvic floor. It is clear that the toxic chemicals to which he had been exposed caused all of this.

Neurotoxicity syndrome is caused by exposure to certain chemicals that affect the brain's ability to communicate with the body. In other words, it is a poisoning of the nervous system. This poisoning can cause brain damage, memory loss, anxiety, depression, impaired mental functioning, limb weakness and numbness, impaired vision, headaches, impaired cognitive functioning, behavioral problems, and even sexual dysfunction.

The human nervous system is one of the most complex systems in nature, and it is responsible for the coordination of thousands of processes, from something as simple as muscle contraction to crying. The center of the nervous system is the brain, and it has over one hundred billion specialized cells called neurons. The central nervous system also dispatches chemical messengers called neurotransmitters.

Research has revealed that the brain has the ability to rewire itself following damage. The brain has a remarkable ability to create new neurons at will, with a little focus and effort. The brain's plasticity continues throughout our lifetime. This involves a variety of processes, including other types of neurons such as glial and vascular cells. Our environment plays an integral role in the process of creating new neural pathways, and this might occur naturally as a result of something like learning.

Many of us take the health of our brains for granted. When our brains are working, we don't pay much attention to it. However, when you suffer from something like toxic metal poisoning, you start to realize how important the health of your brain really is.

According to science, we can now reverse the damage that may have been caused by environmental toxins. Since the brain has the capacity to rewire itself and form new neural pathways, you can improve brain functioning by treating your brain in a healthier manner. For example, the effect of food alone on the brain is so powerful that it can affect your moods.

Much of what we eat contains man-made chemicals. Certain food colors are even made from petroleum, which is not a very pleasant thought. Consuming a lot of sugar and carbohydrates leads to an increase in insulin levels, not to mention the adverse effect of hidden chemicals.

Chemical additives and preservatives are now part of our food, but many of these substances are not meant to be consumed.

In Clint's case, he had to completely change his approach to food. To rid his body of toxins, he had to start feeding his body what it needed to heal.

Metals like arsenic are already present in our soil and water from heavy usage of pesticides, herbicides, animal feed, and power plants. Arsenic is known to cause damage to the peripheral nervous system, and it can cause numbness in the extremities, as well as abnormal EEG readings. Metals like mercury can cause central nervous system damage and brain damage. People with high levels of exposure can even have learning and cognitive difficulties.

Damage to the body's neurological functioning can result in learning disabilities and poor metabolism. Arsenic is extremely damaging to the heart and the cardiovascular system. It may lead to hypertension, anemia, and an increased heart rate.

Heavy metals wreak havoc on the skin, muscles, and hair, and they can cause disruptions in the body's pH levels. This causes rashes and a loss of bone density.

Even low levels of metal in the body can cause a disruption in the endocrine system. The symptoms can vary from aches and pains to hormonal imbalances. Normal functioning of your brain is disrupted by heavy metals. It has been suggested that this kind of interference can accelerate over time, causing the onset of conditions like dementia and Alzheimer's disease.

According to Rudy Silva, a nutritional consultant with a degree in physics from the University of San Jose State, aluminum is associated with Alzheimer's disease. Aluminum was found in high levels in brains of those people who died from Alzheimer's. Because the aluminum industry is quite powerful, any inference that aluminum may cause Alzheimer's likely has been blocked.

Metals can cause all kinds of adverse reactions:

Lead can make one aggressive and hyperactive.
Cadmium can make one aggressive and confused.
Mercury can cause headaches and memory loss.
Aluminum has been linked to dementia and Alzheimer's.

Adding trace minerals along with fresh fruits to the diet can help the body excrete heavy metals.

"Leading scientists recently identified a dozen chemicals as being responsible for widespread behavioral and cognitive problems. But the scope of the chemical dangers in our environment is likely even greater. Children, and the poor are most susceptible to neurotoxic exposure. This cost the U.S. billions of dollars, and immeasurable peace of mind."—James

Hamblin, MD

It is abundantly clear that environmental toxins are not a problem exclusive to welders or those working in toxic or chemical-laden environments.

To process even the most basic information, billions of chemical signals must be constantly carried between neurons. Even when your brain is not actively working, it still uses ten times the number of calories per pound than the rest of your body does.

Chemicals like toluene are used to make nylon and plastic soda bottles; it is also used as a solvent and in certain paints and adhesives. Chlorpyrifos is a pesticide currently utilized on food and nonfood crops. It's classified as highly toxic to birds and freshwater fish, but what does this mean for animals and humans?

Each of our nerve cells is about one-hundredth of a millimeter wide and has to travel its own width twenty-five thousand times merely to move an inch. According to these researchers, a cell can be knocked off course at any point by neurotoxins. There has been a lot of research done on birth defects, but how can this not affect adults as well as children? Chemicals like lead were in gasoline, house paint, and children's toys before scientists realized the extent of the damage it caused. Symptoms of lead poisoning are stomach pain and vomiting, anemia, and even seizures. There are many laws on how lead is used and labeled because of the discovery of its toxic nature.

Chemicals like tetraethyl lead were added to gasoline in 1921, giving it a higher octane rating. The plant that synthesized this chemical was known as "the houses of butterflies" because workers commonly experienced hallucinations that appeared as insects on the skin.

The Toxic Substances Control Act (TSCA) of 1976 is still used today to regulate chemicals, but it has fallen short of its goal. Since the original legislation began, more than twenty thousand new chemicals have entered the marketplace, and only five have been removed. According to these researchers, the legislation is a "toothless, broken piece of legislation."

Chemicals like fluoride are beneficial at low doses but cause tooth and bone lesions at higher amounts. Research has indicated that high fluoride exposure can have a negative effect on brain growth. Mercury, once used in thermometers and barometers, has been found in fish because of coal smokestack emission.

Recent studies have linked fluoride with trace amounts of aluminum. This combination can cause brain and nervous system damage, in addition to an elevated risk of cancer.

Fluoride appears to trigger early-onset brain diseases like Alzheimer's and worsens symptoms in patients already diagnosed with ailments like dementia. Dr. Russell Blaylock infers that adding fluoride to water already containing aluminum can cause destruction of brain cells responsible for memory and learning.

According to Blaylock, fluoride can enhance the toxicity of aluminum for those with aluminum-induced neural degeneration. Aluminum is not considered a heavy metal, although it can be toxic in large or excessive amounts, and it is toxic in even small amounts to the brain. The symptoms of aluminum toxicity can mimic those of Alzheimer's disease and osteoporosis.

Other Symptoms of Aluminum Toxicity

Memory loss

Softening of bones

Aching muscles

Anemia

Headaches

Colic and rickets

Gastrointestinal problems

Speech problems

Aluminum is a naturally occurring element found in our soil, water, and air. It is also used in over-the-counter painkillers and anti-inflammatory products, baking powders, antiperspirants, toothpaste, salt, and beer.

Aluminum may even be the common thread to diseases like Alzheimer's, Parkinson's, and epilepsy. Research indicates aluminum found in everyday items like cookware may significantly contribute to the development of diseases like Alzheimer's and Parkinson's.

Some research has also indicated that high levels of aluminum can play a role in producing certain seizure disorders. Direct evidence has been found in nonhuman primate studies, but we have to ask ourselves if the same thing can be assumed for humans.

We just don't know what kind of long-term damage some of these toxins may cause. In my family's case, it was discovered almost too late to save Clint.

November 2005

I heard the garage door go up. "Mom, I'm home," Clint called from the basement. "I am being sent to Avon to work in the soap plant. They hope I can do it. The work should be easy. I'll be installing valves, screw pipes, steam pipes, poly tubing and bolt up prefab pipe. I'm worried, though. Why can't I get better? I have another appointment with my urologist. He'll probably say I still have a urinary tract infection. But that can't be right. I'm terribly sick! I feel like I haven't slept in weeks."

I sighed. "Don't worry, Clint. You're a big boy. You'll figure it out. Can you eat?"

"No, I'm just too sick."

The urologist continued to treat Clint for urinary tract infections. He decided to keep Clint on Cipro (an antibiotic) continuously.

Clint went to his family physician once or twice a month, asking for help. On November 4, 2005, he received a prescription for Flexeril (muscle relaxant). His back was showing "minimal degenerative changes in the lower spine." Clint had never had any back problems previously. He had always been quite healthy and active. He rode dirt bikes, went camping, and was able to carry large loads—until 2004. Between July 2004 and November 2005, he had done nothing to hurt his back.

He added the horrible symptom rectal bleeding to his growing number of undiagnosed issues.

On November 14, 2005, he returned to the doctor with continuing back pain and was diagnosed with a hernia.

"Mom, all my problems are because I have a hernia," Clint said with a sigh. "The doctor said after I have the hernia fixed, I will feel great. I have an operation scheduled for the thirtieth. I sure hope this works."

"What?" *This is crazy,* I thought. *But who am I to question a doctor?*

"I love you, Clint," I told him as they wheeled him away for the first of what would be many operations. I paced and paced while the doctor fixed a hernia no bigger than a penny.

"I can't believe how much better I feel," Clint told me a couple of days after the operation. His color was better, and he could eat again. I was confused. How could a tiny hernia have caused a year of unexplained sickness? However, I was so relieved to see Clint feeling better that I allowed myself to buy that medical sales pitch. Something still felt off—erroneous.

Clint's newfound wellness, however, didn't last. Less than two weeks later, I heard the words I had heard so many times before. "Mom, I am terribly sick."

December 2005

While Garin decorated our Christmas tree, I went online again to search the internet for information regarding heavy-metal poisoning. In 2005, there was *nothing* about heavy metal. If you look it up today, you'll find page after page of information. Some is useful; most is not. But when I first needed help, there was nothing—nothing at all.

Clint listed his symptoms to me. "My hips are beginning to hurt really badly now. It almost feels like they catch when I walk. My stomach has a twitch down around my pelvic bone on the left side. I'm not sleeping or eating. My skin itches, and I still have this rash. My butt bleeds, and my testicles hurt. It's almost like someone is stomping on them wearing high heels. And above all that, I'm yellow." He sighed and after a moment continued. "I need to pee but can't pee. I am supposed to drink three gallons of water a day, according to the urologist. My knees hurt, and my elbows lock in a bent position when I use my pipe wrenches. I'm dizzy and lightheaded all the time. My vision is occasionally blurry, and I have a nonstop headache." He stopped and thought for a moment. "Do you think any of the prescriptions I'm on are causing any of this? I'm up to about sixteen now. But my doctors say if I stop taking them, they will no longer see me as their patient. Oh, I almost forgot. I'm being moved to Tyson after Christmas."

Garin was disappointed but understanding when I told him we'd have to delay the wedding. I simply couldn't pursue those plans while my son was so ill.

nine

Worsening Symptoms (2006–2007)

January 2006

Clint continued to go to work. He fought through every single miserable day. I worked, as I found relief from all of this by taking on more clients. Even with Garin helping to cover household expenses, Clint's medical costs that weren't covered by insurance were building up too. We were moving faster and faster down that slippery slope.

Clint worked at Tyson through all of January.

February 2006

I heard the garage door go up. "Mom," I heard from a very tired voice in the basement. "I need to eat something I can keep down. Got any ideas?"

Having no answer, I sighed. As a mom, I've always believed it's my job to fix my children's ailments and dilemmas. Lately, I had starting to think I might not be able to fix this one.

In that moment, I decided that I would go to the doctors' appointments with Clint. There had to be something he wasn't saying, or something he wasn't hearing. Otherwise, he'd be getting better.

With dragging steps, Clint climbed up the basement stairs to peer over the ledge above the kitchen sink. He looked like death. Like a person who couldn't get out of bed. I could tell, just by looking at him, how deeply tired he was.

"I'm going to work at a drywall plant in Roanoke tomorrow. My buddies will be there, so I'll have help to get through my days and get to the doctors. I'm a little scared, though. The work will be off the ground, and the medication I take affects my balance. Plus, my hips are locking up more and more. I hope I don't fall or anything."

Oh, my God, I don't want to hear this, I thought, cringing as horrible images raced through my mind.

"It's new construction. They're adding on to the plant. No chemical exposure," he said. "I'm going to lie on the cold basement floor. It's the only place I can go to relieve some of this pain in my groin. Damn, I hurt all over."

From then on, I went with Clint to the doctors' visits. The doctors and their staff didn't care for that. They would say things to degrade me or to try to discourage me from attending the visits. For some reason with each new doctor, Clint and I always had a renewed sense of hope. I really felt like my accompanying Clint to his appointments would help. I searched for ideas on the internet. I printed articles that matched his symptoms, with medical clues to help solve this mystery.

When I tried to share my research, this is what I was told: "You are not a doctor. You are not qualified to diagnose your son's illness. You need to stay off the internet. You need to do your job, and let us do ours." Each doctor shut me down. They made me feel small and stupid. I knew I was right. But right was not good enough in the ego world of medicine. A degree with PhD is what mattered to them. I was *just* a *mom*. "What do people do when doctors don't listen?" I kept asking myself.

"This is Clint's problem; it's not his *mother's* place to help him. He needs to take care of this on his own," they'd say.

All of a sudden, I was added to the medical notes, as if Clint and I were codependents. They treated us like we had mental issues or as if we were drug seekers, or both.

I understood why Clint was not able to communicate with his doctors. Doctors don't communicate or connect with their patients when their patients are mysteriously sick or don't fit into perfectly laid-out, prequalified insurance codes that identify accepted illnesses.

Clint was diagnosed with prostatitis (inflammation of the prostate gland), which is often brought on by infection.

April–June 2006

"Try to get some sleep, Clint. Tomorrow will be another rough day." I just wanted to cry. Clint was going to have *another* procedure. This procedure would be a cystoscopy, so the doctor could examine the lining of his bladder and urethra, and urethral dilation.

"How are you feeling?" I asked my son as he woke up from surgery later that day.

"Okay," he said drowsily. "Once the pain medication wears off and the sugar water clears out of my blood, I know I will hurt again. I wish I could just stay here."

After the procedure, we went home. Ten days later, Clint was in serious pain again.

Clint continued to work at the drywall plant, but he was missing a lot of time because of all of his aliments. A hard worker, he continued going to work as much as he possibly could. Every morning, he had to stop halfway to the job site and throw up from the pain.

I took a swim kickboard (a Styrofoam float children use in swimming pools) and cut out a U-shape in the center to try to get the pressure off his testicles when he sat in the car.

It didn't help. Nothing helped. He lived in constant pain. His hips and testicles hurt badly, but he just kept on working.

Days turned into weeks and weeks into months, and Clint continued to struggle. When home, he spent most of his time lying spread-eagle on the cold basement floor. The muscles in his stomach quivered, and his body shook from pain.

I didn't understand; why didn't a single doctor take a few minutes and look at *all* the symptoms? We had a dermatologist for his skin rash and a spinal doctor for his back. We had a urologist for his prostate problem and a general doctor for ... well, no good reason. We had a psychologist for his depression and pain and an eye doctor who just kept saying, "I have never seen a film like this grow over someone's eye before."

Looking back, I realize that we didn't have any healers. What we did have was a growing stack of bills leading directly to the poorhouse.

Having been diagnosed with prostatitis, by June 2006, Clint was seeing his fifth urologist. Each one said the same thing. "This will take time. I need you to promise me six months. If you give me six months, I will make you better, but you have to follow my instructions to the letter. Take the prescriptions I provide for you."

Clint did exactly what he was told for five separate urologists. In the end, they told him there was nothing more they could do. They blamed depression and anxiety for all of his symptoms. The urologist that treated Clint in June 2006 decided that his urethra needed to be stretched—not just once but many times. He decided Clint needed more medication added to his already-long list of prescriptions.

Clint was taking Flomax and Avodart at the same time. None of the doctors took the time to see how these drugs affected Clint's liver and adrenal glands. His liver was diagnosed in 2004 as jaundiced, but that didn't stop the doctors from prescribing medication after medication. After six months, when the drugs didn't work, each urologist told Clint there was nothing more he or she could do.

Clint's symptoms now included the following:

> Constant flu-like symptoms
> Joints locking up
> Chest pain
> Ankle pain and toe cramping
> Headache
> Skin yellowing
> Translucent teeth with a silver shine; swollen gums
> Night sweats
> Ear bleeding
> Inability to sleep
> Rectal bleeding
> Morning sickness
> Extreme hip joint pain
> Constant soft-tissue pain
> Intestinal dysfunction
> Boggy, spongy prostate
> Urinary tract spasms
> Testicular pain and inflammation with inability to urinate
> Extremely swollen lymph nodes throughout his entire body

It was June 2006 when Clint called me, sobbing. He was in his truck in the parking lot, outside urologist number five's office. I remember where I was working. I remember that day, with posttraumatic flashback agony, like it was yesterday.

"Mom," he cried, "I am in so much pain. I left work and drove to my urologist, hoping he would see me in this horrible condition and finally understand what I am experiencing. I walked in the office, and his nurses said since I didn't have an appointment, I had to leave—now. I told them about my pain in my testicles and stomach. They didn't care. They called the police on me. They told me to go to the emergency room. How many times have we gone there? How many times did they profile us as pain-med seekers and tell me I had to make an appointment with my doctor for help? I know, you know, that this is their way of pushing me away. There's nowhere for me to go. I have knives being driven into my balls. I cannot stand. I cannot sit. I cannot lie down to get out of pain. I am throwing up; the pain is so intense. Why can't somebody see this and help? What am I going to do? They pushed me out the door and locked it shut. The cops are on their way." He just kept crying in pain. "Something is inside of me, eating me alive. What is it?"

The sun was shining, and the world was hot and busy. People were having picnics and summer fun. Clint's and my world just kept getting worse. I hated the sun. I hated the sounds of children outside, playing. I wanted it to be rainy and dark. My head was rainy and dark, and the sunny outside world made me feel worse. Nothing about my life was able to make me forget this world of never-ending pain with no answers in sight. It seemed like the only way for it to end was Clint's death. Clint wanted to die. He just couldn't stop the fight.

Clint is a fighter. I am a warrior. I tried to calm him down. I told him to breathe. Get a drink of water. By this time, he was drinking five gallons of water a day. He was told to do this by each urologist he saw. He was on urologist number five, and the gallons of water to drink each day matched.

Clint sat in his truck, and we talked for a little while. By this time his pelvic-floor muscles were failing from the metals attacking his soft tissue. His brain was sending out so many soldiers to fight the metals that the inflammation in his body was causing extreme pain.

However, at this time neither of us understood what was wrong. There was still no information on the internet about over body burden and related cellular death. I believed then, and still do today, that his doctors knew. They just would not cross over the forbidden bridge into the land of truth in medicine. Our Western world of doctors still has to stay the course. The course is, "There is no such thing as heavy-metal poisoning."

I cried. Clint cried. We had nowhere to go. Nowhere to turn. We were still stuck in the pain-box mystery.

Clint went back to work. That is what he did. He pushed through. He went on, no matter what came his way. My day was a disaster filled with uncontrolled anger and fear. Clint's day was filled with pain.

That's when I called the doctor and made a huge mistake. I asked the doctor, "Do you think he could be poisoned?"

We were immediately asked to leave, and Clint was sent back to his general doctor. This brought another problem, as Dr. Hanes no longer wanted to deal with us either.

July 2006

At that point, Dr. Hanes shoved us off to a different doctor within the practice.

"Mom," Clint said, "I'm going to stop going to my doctor. I'm going to see a female doctor. Weird, I know. It's okay. Dr. Hanes wasn't very nice. First, he said I was sick from eating fish from the lakes in Parkersburg. Then, he said I was sick because I rode my dirt bike through mud puddles. Then, he said I was sick because I must be having sex with multiple women. Then, he said I must be sick because I must be having sex with multiple men." Clint looked exasperated.

His new doctor took all kinds of notes. Oh my goodness, she seemed extremely interested in Clint. She was bound and determined to help him. She emphatically believed he had been poisoned. She just knew it.

Dr. Corey explained to us that she was working on the DuPont Teflon case in Pennsylvania. This doctor was so interested in Clint's history that she took extensive notes on all of his places of work. She wanted to know what he did, how long he did those tasks at each location, and what chemicals he suspected he'd come in contact. Hindsight makes me think that she was gathering information from Clint to use for her own case associated with DuPont. Once she finished using Clint for her own project, she stopped seeing Clint and referred him back to Dr. Hanes. Horrible for a doctor to exploit a terminally ill patient for her own ego. Dr. Hanes, again, didn't want him either. Eventually, Clint lost hope in that practice, and sometime later, we stopped our visits entirely.

I'm angry as I wonder who Dr. Corey was working for as she used Clint for her case study. Was she wearing a white hat? I have such a negative attitude regarding such things that I feel probably not. Then I console myself with the thought that she lost, and there's a little *yippee* in my head.

An article on Bloomberg.com states, "DuPont Co. was found liable for a man's testicular cancer in the second lawsuit to go to trial in 3,500 lawsuits over a toxic Teflon chemical found in Ohio and West Virginia waters, for which spinoff Chemours Co. had agreed to bear the cost."

"Don't worry, Clint. I'm working on it," I told him. I was worrying enough for both of us, spending hours and hours searching for information on heavy-metal poisoning. In 2006, there still wasn't any information.

We began seeing a new urologist. This led to the same diagnosis as the previous doctors had given. More of the same included the following:

Boggy prostate of unknown cause
Urinary frequency with inability to void
Multiple symptoms of unrelated causes
Depression and anxiety

Once again, this doctor would not answer my questions about the arsenic and bilirubin levels in his blood tests in 2004. He refused to order any more blood tests regarding those results so long ago. Why? Again, the doctor refused to listen.

After hearing the words I'd heard a few dozen times—"Clint is mentally depressed and anxious. His pains are psychosomatic, and I can't help him. I'm sorry"—I finally asked, "What do you think came first? The never-ending pain that caused the depression and anxiety, or the depression and anxiety that caused the pain? Because I can tell you this: he was not depressed or anxious in 2004 when all of this started!"

The doctor shook his head. "You and Clint are too dependent on one another, Peggy. You both need psychiatric help." His face was calm. To be honest, by this point he was probably right. After everything we'd been through, we probably had been driven a little mad. We were finished. Nothing had worked, and Clint was sicker than ever.

Although Garin remained supportive, one day he interrupted a conversation between my son and me with a remark to Clint. "You really shouldn't bother your mother with these things! You're an adult. At the very least, surely you could make your own doctor appointments."

Although the intrusion angered me, I ignored the comment, and Clint followed my lead. We concluded our discussion and went on with our day.

But later, I thought about it and decided that perhaps if Garin could not understand how I felt about this, the wedding should be not just delayed but canceled altogether. Thus was the seed of discord planted between Garin and me. Battle lines had been drawn. Before we had even gotten married, the honeymoon was over.

I decided to try one more urologist. Once again, I was convinced that a doctor, this time in the person of Dr. Barstow, was going to save my son. I could not have been more wrong. His final diagnosis was the worst of all. The words "pelvic-floor disease" rolled off the doctor's tongue, devoid of any compassion whatsoever.

Pelvic-floor disease describes the failure of muscles that keep all of a person's organs in place. Everything on the inside wants to fall out. It's a life sentence of pain.

"You have pelvic-floor disease. It's chronic. You will never get any better because there is no cure. Unfortunately, there isn't any medication that completely alleviates the pain. I recommend that you find a support group and a pain-management doctor. You're going to need a team of doctors and a support group to help you manage your symptoms."

Feeling as if I had rocketed headfirst into a brick wall, I looked at the doctor, dazed and defeated. "Will you be part of this team?" I asked in a small, sad voice. "Can you help us do this? And can you point us in the direction of a support group? Do you have other patients with this disease that we can join with to make a support group?"

He looked at me sternly. "I'm too busy to deal with things like this. You have to find your team of doctors and look for your own support group."

"What the hell do you think we've been doing since 2004?" I asked furiously. My voice was no longer quiet and sad. "I'm convinced there aren't any doctors left in this world. They're bottom-feeders who take our money while pretending to be doctors! Instead of conferring with one another, you send each other little notes about your shared patients. But do any of you even read them? Never once have I seen a doctor read or refer to those notes! When we go to our appointments, you all ask the same questions over and over and over again. You are one sad, sorry group of arrogant people, if you ask me!" When we walked out of that office, both Clint and I had tears in our eyes.

I called to cancel dinner plans with Garin, and when he protested, I told him tiredly, "Consider the engagement off, Garin. You're free. I've got bigger fish to fry." Without waiting for his response, I disconnected the call. He deserved better from me, but I didn't have anything better to give him at the time.

Sick days rolled into pain-filled weeks and months. Clint struggled to stay alive, and I struggled, desperately searching for answers and ideas to ease his pain. Our past lives disappeared, and neither of us could remember what that past was like. We both forgot how to laugh. I lost contact with most of my friends. When I did try to go out for a short time, I could not stop worrying. I cannot remember much of my life during those years. All I remember is the battle to find answers as the death clock kept ticking in my brain. I cannot remember Clint's birthday. I cannot remember Christmas. My memory is empty except for pain and suffering. If it was a sunny day, I wished it was raining. It was a terribly dark time.

I spent all winter gathering information and organizing Clint's medical records. I tried to find answers about pelvic-floor disease.

March 2007

While searching for information about pelvic-floor disease, I found a local physical rehabilitation center for trauma patients called Diamond Rehab Center. I contacted Diamond to see if they treated pelvic-floor disease. They did, so I began the intake process to get therapy for Clint.

Insurance only gives a person twenty physical therapy visits a year. To correct most ailments, this is hardly enough. But once again, I accepted the fact that I would be paying out of pocket for this care.

I also found Dr. Noel Sampson in Los Angeles and read his book, *The Pelvic Battleground.* It described *some* of Clint's pain perfectly. I decided to email Dr. Sampson. Unbelievably, he responded to my emails. We had several email conversations.

A couple of months later, he called my cell phone from LA. I will never forget that Tuesday morning. When he told me he wanted to talk to Clint, I gave him Clint's cell phone number.

This was the first of many conversations with him. Dr. Sampson wanted me to fly Clint to Los Angeles so he could treat him. Clint emphatically said he couldn't fly or go that far from home. His pain was so intense that he would never be able to sit in an airplane. He threw up every time he ate. He was so weak that the trip was not possible.

That being the case, Dr. Sampson wanted Clint to go to a specialty clinic associated with Johns Hopkins Hospital. He knew Dr. Platt, the director of urology there. He said he would make the contact for Clint and begin the intake process.

By this time, Clint was already going to the Diamond Rehab Center two times a week for pelvic-floor therapy. Therapy doesn't work overnight, and we understood that. Clint would go in the morning before his shift at the drywall plant.

He was still quite sick, and it seemed like his hips were getting worse by the minute. We went to orthopedic doctors, but they couldn't find anything wrong with his hips. Repeatedly, orthopedists referred him back to urology. We had beaten that to death already; we couldn't keep going to urologists.

Clint continued working hard on the pelvic-floor exercises, hoping that would bring him the relief he was seeking. In the meantime, I worked on getting him into the Johns Hopkins Hospital's clinic. Waiting time for an appointment was eight weeks.

The drive to the appointment to see Dr. Platt was horrible. Clint was in so much pain, it made the five-hour drive seemed like a three-day trip. Then, after the appointment, we had to drive five hours to come home. By this time, Clint looked like a serious drug abuser. Dr. Sampson had said that the only drug that would help pelvic-floor pain was Valium. He would have prescribed Valium immediately if Clint was his patient. Dr. Platt would have prescribed Valium if she was his official doctor. But neither could give Clint what they thought could help him!

Clint had drawers and drawers full of narcotics that he didn't take because they didn't work. However, no doctor in Charleston would prescribe Valium. It was considered too dangerous. And for some reason, all the oxy drugs that he was prescribed (with other assorted narcotics) were just fine. My *nice mom* attitude was gone. I was done being nice.

Garin, on the other hand, began to seem *too* nice. He was kind, supportive, and irritatingly unflappable. But as I increasingly grew into a frenzy to try to save Clint, Garin politely distanced himself from the process.

June 2007

By June, Clint was going to Diamond for pelvic-floor therapy and to a chiropractor for his back and testicular pain. He was occasionally seeing his general practitioner, Dr. Corey, who was working on the DuPont case. We were still hoping that she was one of the good guys. It was only out of desperation that we kept going to see her. She would not prescribe the much-needed Valium that Dr. Sampson recommended.

In order to get Valium, I decide Clint needed to go to a sleep clinic. He was in too much pain to sleep, so maybe a doctor at the clinic would prescribe that magic pain pill for Clint.

The doctor with the sleep clinic became very interested in Clint's story. He understood heavy-metal poisoning, but it was clear that the topic was off limits. He knew of Dr. Sampson, and he understood Clint's situation without saying it. He prescribed Valium, which gave Clint a few hours here and there without pain.

Clint became a hoarder of his Valium supply. He didn't take them every day for fear that when he desperately needed them, he would be out. He was very cautious with them and used them as his fallback.

"Clint, how are you feeling today?" I asked. Knowing I wouldn't hear an answer I liked, I still had to ask. As his mother, I needed to know.

"Not too good, Mom," he said. "But at least if it gets too bad, I can take a Valium. Sometimes I can even sleep a few hours at night."

Garin and I were just sharing living space. The loving relationship was over. Clint's situation was one of twenty-four/seven nonstop pain. I didn't even have five minutes to spend on anyone besides my son.

Garin resented Clint—and Clint was angry that Garin was still living with us but not supporting me emotionally. I had enough to deal with. The decision about Garin's and my future had to wait.

One afternoon while I was working, my cell phone rang. At a glance, I saw Clint was calling, and I was immediately nervous about answering. I knew it would be something horrible. I was starting to feel like I couldn't bear another minute of his pain.

"Mom, I have to tell you something. Just in case I don't make it out of this mess," he said. My gut flip-flopped. "I am standing on a slanted roof about twenty feet in the air. My left hip is locked in place. My right hip is shaking, and I can't move at all. I may not get out of this. I love you. Thanks for all of your help. I know you did the best you could. I wish I could understand why any of this is happening."

My heart was pounding, my hands were sweating, and my head was spinning. I struggled to get my thoughts in order. I needed to be strong for Clint. "Clint," I said as calmly as I could muster, "take a deep breath. Breathe. Breathe." I heard him breathing. "Calmly try to sit down. Breathe in and out. Take it easy. Take your time. Just bend down."

"Okay, I'm breathing. I'm trying," he said. I waited. I heard him cry out in pain. "It hurts!" He groaned and sat down. I talked him through the pain as his hips began to move. He climbed down off the roof and came home.

That was the day I decided he was through taking all his current medications. They weren't making a difference now and never had. Not one helped, with the singular exception of the Valium, which most doctors wouldn't prescribe to him. For some reason, Valium was more controlled than Oxycontin, Percocet, or oxycodone, more controlled than any of the other drugs Clint was prescribed.

The garage door went up. I heard Clint enter. "Oh, Mom, I'm sorry about today. I guess I panicked," he said, tired and downtrodden. "I really thought I was going to die. I almost wish I had. I'm so tired of being in pain all the time."

I felt like a failure. *Come on, think … There has to be an answer. I have to find the answer.* Then I began to feel guilty. Clint had been sick, really sick, in excruciating pain. He was giving up. *How can I keep pushing and pushing when I am not the one living in his hell?*

I wanted to cry but was afraid that would make Clint feel guilty. We didn't need two guilty people. He came upstairs, and I told him something I hadn't yet confided about the hopelessness I felt. It might be time for him to just give up. "I understand how you feel, and I will respect any decision that you make regarding your future."

"I'm sorry for ruining your life, Mom!" he said with a sob.

I hugged him, and when his tears subsided, I told him, "Life is just this way, son. There are no guarantees of anything—just life 'til death. That's all we get."

At just that moment, Garin came in the front door with a hearty shout. "I'm home and hungry, Peg! If you haven't started supper yet, want to go out tonight?"

I could have throttled him.

July 2007

In all fairness, Garin's concerns truly were all about me. He continued helping with the cooking and mowing and other practical matters, with a constant focus on supporting my well-being. As the medical bills skyrocketed, Garin assumed a greater proportion of the household bills without complaint. However, this was not *his* son. It was always like Garin was on the outside, looking in.

The engagement ring, which I had taken off and put on the dresser many months before, remained where it was. The accusing piece of jewelry sat twinkling on its own little plot of undusted real estate.

As time went on, resentments grew between Garin and Clint. I was often caught in disputes over things as simple as who should have wiped off the counter or what parking place in the driveway was theirs. One day, they even bickered over whether or not Miracle Whip was too sweet to use on BLT sandwiches. Garin's request for Clint to move his truck might be met by a growl and "You're not my father."

Clint's comment that someone shouldn't leave his briefcase and stacks of files in the den might be countered with "Someone ought to let go of his mother's apron strings."

I told Garin I simply didn't think it was going to work out between us. He did not argue with me, though at times I would wish he'd fight harder to keep us together.

Eventually, he bought a house in a neighboring community and moved out. We remained close, and as far as I know, neither of us dated anyone else before we got the real diagnosis. But I'm getting ahead of myself.

August 2007

"Make sure you have everything," I said as Clint was gathering his things to go to Baltimore. We were both expecting great things to happen.

Having stopped taking all of the prescription drugs, Clint had found that nothing had changed, for good or ill. Clint had tried to talk with Dr.

Platt about heavy-metal poisoning. She, like everyone else, lived the Western medical denial game and said something dismissive about government regulations and there being no proof that he was suffering from heavy-metal toxicity.

So Clint went to Baltimore, playing by their rules. We were learning.

While Clint was in Baltimore, I would be going to Tallahassee for Sarah's graduation from law school. What a mess. The previous fall, Clint had bought a ticket to Tallahassee too, hoping to be well. Instead, he was worse off than ever and on his way to spend two weeks in Baltimore.

"I'm sorry I can't drive you there," I told him. He looked so weak and tired I almost broke down and called Garin for help. Almost. "We'll talk while you drive so I know you are okay … Well, as okay as you can be. You have the room information and all of the clinic's paperwork, right?" My maternal instinct never went away.

"Yes, Mom," he said, with hope brightening his voice. "I'll be fine. I'm going to get better. They're going to repair my pelvic floor!"

I sighed, gave him a hug, and sent him on his way. I waved as I watched him drive away, knowing it would be a very painful trip for him. I over-thought for a little while but had to pull myself together. I had a graduation celebration in six days. There were bags to pack and a plane to catch.

One day at a time, I told myself. *When will this ever end? I need a break—and Clint needs a pain-free day followed by a full night's sleep.*

About two hours later, I got a phone call from Clint. "Mom, I'm halfway there."

I had been pacing since he left, trying to pack my suitcase and get into a happy graduation frame of mind.

"Good. How are you feeling?" I asked. Part of me wished I could stop asking and stop dreading the answer.

"Not too bad," he said. "I hurt, like always. But it could be worse. I wish I was going to Tallahassee with you. Tell my sister how sorry I am."

"I will," I replied. "Don't worry. Just focus on feeling better. She understands why you can't make it."

On Wednesday, I left for Florida. Clint was on his third day of therapy. "Mom," he said, "I think this is working. I already feel better—only a tiny bit but better. I think I need to stay here until I'm healthy."

"I will work on that after the graduation," I promised. I would be in Florida for a week after the graduation, staying with my grandchild and "grand-dog," house-sitting while Sarah and Mark enjoyed Hawaii on a long overdue vacation. I anticipated having some downtime to call around and see what I could do to help Clint.

The Monday after the graduation, I got to work.

First, I contacted the clinic in Baltimore to see if they would continue to work with Clint if I could move him there temporarily. They said no.

Then I made a lot of phone calls. I called every physical therapist I could find on the internet. I pleaded with and begged each one to learn the pelvic-floor protocol. No one was interested in helping.

Athens, West Virginia, is a little over an hour from my house. When I called a hospital located there to talk to their physical therapy department, someone was finally willing to learn about pelvic-floor rehabilitation!

I called the Johns Hopkins clinic and talked with Dr. Platt to let her know that I had found someone near us that was willing to learn the technique. That's exactly what they told me to do—to find someone close to home and let them "practice" on Clint.

Through one of the many telephone conversations that I had with strangers, I learned about a woman in Charleston who owned a pelvic-floor therapy clinic. I called Kara Norberg, a pelvic-floor therapist. In 2007 when I contacted her, this type of rehabilitation was just beginning. I got the impression that Kara did not get respect from the urologists she supported. Pelvic-floor dysfunction in men was not yet understood. Western medicine has identified reasons why women have pelvic-floor disease: childbirth, endometriosis, and urinary tract infections. In the absence of significant data regarding male pelvic-floor dysfunction, Western medicine defaults to mental disorder as the explanation. The male patient must have unresolved childhood issues or be suffering from depression and anxiety.

What came first? I asked the question again. I was certain. *The pelvic-floor pain began after he worked on the arsenic-cleaning water machine. On the heels of that came depression and anxiety.*

"Hello, Kara," I greeted her. "Do you have a few minutes to talk to me? I have a thirty-four-year-old son who has been diagnosed with pelvic-floor disease. He is at Johns Hopkins Hospital now. I asked if I could rent an apartment in Baltimore for him so he could continue there, and they said no. The specialty clinic only sees residents of Baltimore as regular patients. Residents of other cities must go home and find their own therapists. Problem is, there aren't any around, and the clinic won't budge about helping him. Clint is seeing great results, so we can't stop now. Would you be willing to help?"

Kara was very calm and had a take-charge attitude. "I only treat women," she explained. "I'm sorry, but the few men I have treated just didn't get well. My studio is not really made for men and women. Because of the embarrassing nature of the recovery process for pelvic floor, women don't want men around when they are recovering. I am very sorry."

I was frustrated and in a bad place emotionally. I felt like we were close to recovery, if we could just get some help. "I understand," I told her. I sighed, and asked again. "Won't you please just try? Once you see him, you'll understand how much he needs your help. A woman in Athens has agreed to learn the protocol. Maybe you could train her. I would pay you, if you'd be willing."

There was a pause in the conversation, during which I heard every beat of my heart.

"I'm always looking for people who want to learn what I do. That may work," she said finally.

"Can I send Clint to see you, then?" I asked.

"I don't have an opening for more than a month," she replied.

"That's okay. Clint can go to Athens and begin to show that therapist what he learned at Johns Hopkins while we wait for you." I was beginning to see a light at the end of the tunnel.

When I called Clint later, I asked, "How are you doing? Finding anything fun to do between therapy sessions?"

"Oh, Mom," he said, "I am feeling much better! This works! This is what I need. I need to stay here and continue with this treatment. Guess what? I felt so good last night I actually went to a baseball game! Can you believe that? My hips still hurt. This doesn't help that. But oh my God, the pelvic pain has let up at least 25 percent!"

I convinced the clinic to continue treating Clint for one more week. When he came home, he looked much better. He still had pain—but nothing as bad as before. We knew we were headed in the right direction. He could feel it and see it! I had hope again.

Clint went back to work and somehow drove to Athens two days a week. It was not easy. Determined to get well, he was working thirty miles away from home and then driving about forty-five miles to Athens.

Finally, a month later, Clint met Kara. As I had hoped, she immediately recognized the seriousness of Clint's situation. She agreed to begin treating him. It was the one and only positive thing to happen for Clint in four years.

September 2007

I heard the garage door go up. "Mom," Clint called from the basement. "I'm moving back to Tyson's food plant. Good thing because winter's coming. I don't want to work outside in the cold. I'm too exhausted for that."

Clint continued to go to the sleep clinic. He saw Kara two times a week. He did his pelvic-floor exercises every chance he had and continued to hoard and protect his Valium. Kara had a pain-management doctor that she thought could help, and Clint began seeing him.

Neither Kara's nor Dr. Payne's visits were covered by insurance. Neither was the sleep clinic. Money was pouring out of my budget faster than ever before. I picked up more freelance clients to cover the expenses. Clint was finally making positive progress, so the money spent was well worth it. I continued to make personal sacrifices, as any mother would. Soon I was out of money, out of time, and too exhausted to care about myself. I stopped going to the gym.

December 2007

"Goodbye, Clint," I said as he dropped me off at the airport the week before Christmas. "I'll see you in ten days. Keep up the hard work. It's paying off!"

"Yep, you're right! I love you, Mom. Bye."

On Christmas Day, my cell phone rang. I looked down to see that it was Clint. Afraid that he was hurting again, I answered with a touch of dread. Honestly, that is how I answered the phone every time I saw his number. All phone calls from Clint had become more conversations of the same: pain, pain, and more pain.

"Mom, I was just fired," he said.

"What? Why?"

"They know I'm not well. They think it's their fault. I thought they were working with me because they cared. But after talking to a few of my friends at work, I am not so sure. They've been talking to the guys in the field. There are other guys who worked at ULTRA who are sick. I wasn't working for this company when I was at ULTRA, but I'm fired either way. They said I missed too many days, and I guess I can't blame them; I've missed a lot of days. No argument there. Maybe it's okay. I need some time off anyway. I need to get healthy. This pelvic-floor rehab is working. Maybe if I keep working harder, I'll get well."

"I'm good with that if you are," I told him. "Take care of yourself. I'll be home in a few days, and we'll figure this out. I promise."

Ten

Hip Injections (2008–2009)

January–August 2008

Clint was very sick. His hips were a mess. The pelvic-floor situation was improving, but he still could not sleep. He could not eat without throwing up. His muscles would tense up and pulse just below the skin. His skin turned a sickly shade of brownish gray, and his eyes grew dull. He was having trouble hearing. Irritable, he had a quick-to-snap attitude. I had not seen this in him since his teen days. He was just burned out.

Dr. Payne—the pain doctor Kara had suggested—began injecting "self-harvested" PRP (platelet rich plasma) cells into Clint's hips. At $175 a visit, this was expensive. But again, it seemed to work, so it had to happen. Anything that gave us a ray of hope was worth every penny. I went to many of these visits, and I truly believe Dr. Payne knew Clint's real diagnosis.

His staff told me that Clint should get out of the pipe-fitting business. They constantly commented how bad it was for him and for his disease. They would say things like, "He must avoid dangerous exposure." They were careful not to mention poisoning, but they made it clear that they did know. Dr. Payne, just like all the other doctors, wouldn't say the words *heavy-metal poisoning*. The phrase was a four-letter word in the medical community.

Once again, I attempted to research heavy-metal poisoning. Still, I came up short. Dr. Payne just kept shooting up Clint with the plasma cells. Clint would feel better for a few weeks and then need more injections. Both of his hips needed shots. Dr. Payne was more than happy to continue this expensive therapy. Were we just a cash cow to him?

"Moo, moo, moo," I muttered, writing yet another check.

Clint's needs continued, so I found more work. Dr. Payne did more PRP cell injections.

Clint's pelvic floor therapist was a gift from heaven. Kara told him from the very beginning that she had never helped a man before. "I haven't met a man who will work hard enough or long enough to get well," she said. "It's just more difficult for a man." Actually, very few women are determined enough to see it through. Clint is different. He worked, and worked, and worked. He wanted to get better. He needed to get better.

His hard work was paying off. The pelvic-floor pain was subsiding. Some of his other symptoms were letting up along with it. He was still in pain. Fortunately, the level of pain was dropping. The pain in his hips continued, though, and he still rarely slept. But everything else was letting up.

"Mom, Mom, Mom!" I woke up to his panicked voice. It was the middle of the night, and Clint was standing next to my bed. "I am so sick I can't sleep. I'm scared. What if I never get better? I can't keep this up. I'm just so sick of being sick. I want my life back!" Clint was cracking under the pressure of his illness.

I frowned. I wanted to help him but didn't know how.

"Clint, please just go back to bed. Try to rest." I tried to sound positive. "How's the Valium supply? You can always take one of those. They always help."

"I can't keep taking them. I don't want to become addicted ... and I have to save them for the really bad times."

"Progress is slow, but your hard work is paying off," I whispered. "You've been able to sleep for a few hours a night and have been able to eat a little bit without throwing up. The pelvic-floor pain is subsiding. Some of your other symptoms are letting up too. I know the pain in your hips continues. But everything else is letting up. Things are not good—but they're better than they have been!"

"Mom, I hurt!" he insisted, demanding of me something I longed to give but was unable. Since his birth, as with all my children, I was the healer. I always found solutions to their problems. Serious thoughts of doubt were repeating in my brain. As a warrior, I knew these thoughts would cause defeat. Victory is a mental game. To win, I had to think like a winner, not a quitter. Yet I had nothing in my mental arsenal to give me that power.

"Clint, I can't help you right now. I have to work in the morning. I have to be able to think. Please, you can't do this to me during the day and then all night long too. Please, I know you're sick. I know you're tired. I'm tired too. I need you to stay strong. Stay the course. Keep working with Kara. I make the money; you do the work. Remember?"

"Okay, I'm sorry," he said, defeated. "The nights are the worst. It's so scary, and I'm just in my own head all night long. My brain won't stop. I can't lie on my hips. My back hurts. My head hurts. I want to die. Why can't I just die?"

I watched as his bent, broken-down body left my room. The outside light made his silhouette look ghostly. He walked like an old man. Then I couldn't stop thinking. I decided that first thing in the morning, I would try harder to find answers. Clint was counting on me.

As many nights' before, I heard the garage door go up and knew Clint was pacing outside, trying to get relief from his pain. I must have dozed off while I waited for him to come back inside. Sometime in the darkness, I heard the garage door close, waking me from my unintended nap. I heard his feet shuffle into the bathroom downstairs. I heard the toilet flush again. How many times was that tonight? All night long, he tried to pee with no relief.

But with all that said, he *was* getting a little better. His suffering had gone on for such a long time; a little improvement was not enough. As I did every morning, I tiptoed out of bed and into the shower.

Be quiet. Be very quiet. If he is sleeping, don't wake him. Pretend this isn't happening for a moment! Pretend this is not another day of the unknown, not another day of watching my son die. The shower will make me feel better. Get into the shower. Breathe. Stop thinking. Just breathe. I got in the shower and tried to let the warm water relax my tense muscles.

As I turned off the shower, I heard the downstairs toilet flush. Another painful day had begun.

"Mom!" Clint called for me. I knew he had lain for hours on the basement floor. "I didn't sleep one minute. Not one. I just want to die. I feel horrible!"

I sighed. *Go away!* I wanted to scream. *Go the hell away!* Instead, I said, "It will be okay; you're getting better. Yesterday was a little better than Christmas last year. Remember how awful you felt then? Don't forget to recognize the baby steps you're taking. Go see Kara today. It's working. When do you go see Dr. Payne again?"

As I did every weekday morning, I gathered up my computer and lunch and headed off to work. Clint stood in the hallway leading into his bathroom. He looked like death. As usual, he followed me to my car, crying in pain, telling me about his horribly long, painful night. He stood there watching as I drove away.

How long until he would start to take those pills he had left over from all the operations? How long until he would decide enough was enough and kill himself? I drove away, watching him grow increasingly smaller in my rearview mirror.

Clint was tough. He kept going to Kara. I would hear him all night long, shuffling to and from the bathroom. He moaned in pain as he lay on the concrete floor. I heard him doing the pelvic-floor exercises throughout the night.

"If I can't sleep, I may as well do the exercises," he explained to me.

All of his work was paying off. In June, Clint started to feel better. Some days the urinary issue was barely there. Some days his hips didn't hurt. Some nights he could sleep for a few hours.

Dr. Payne kept doing the PRP treatments. That's all he would do, though. I was starting to think something was wrong with his plan. It only helped Clint for a little while. It wasn't a permanent solution.

September 2008

I heard the garage go up. "Mom!" Clint yelled excitedly. "Kara can't believe it. She says she has never seen anything like this. She says she's never seen anyone work like I have to beat pelvic floor, and my pelvic muscles are functioning!" Then his voice changed. "That's the good news. The bad news is, she can't figure out why I have to pee all the time. She wants me to go to a different urologist to see if anything has changed." He sighed. "Why bother with them? They are useless!" With that, he shuffled down the hall into the bathroom.

The next day we made an appointment with another urologist. As in the past, we had to wait six weeks to get an appointment. The new doctor decided that Clint's urethra had collapsed and needed to be stretched every day. Clint was taught how to catheterize himself, which allowed him to pee without pushing and undoing all of his pelvic-floor rehab. Clint continued to do this while he faithfully did his pelvic-floor exercises. He was terrified that the pelvic-floor pain could return. But overall, catheterization seemed to help. Some of the urinating issues let up. His yellow skin became more normal. He was coming back to life in front of my eyes!

Toward the end of the month, Garin talked me into going out to dinner and dancing. It was a beautiful evening. With Clint feeling better, I danced and laughed. "Maybe everything is going to be all right," I said.

"Everything is all right," Garin assured me. With all my heart, I wanted to believe him.

October 2008

I was in the kitchen when Clint yelled from the basement, "Mom! I'm going back to work. I'm over all of this. I'm not perfectly healthy yet, but I'm going back anyway. I need to work, Mom. I start in two weeks working at a paper mill in Clarksburg. The drive isn't going to be fun. The job will suck. It's a shutdown. But I have to start somewhere. I need my life back. So I'm going to start by going to work."

Please don't do this. It's too early, I pleaded silently, knowing I couldn't say this to Clint out loud. He needed to feel like he had some control over his own life. He needed to do this for his own sanity.

"Great!" I called back. "At least it's not too far from home or too far from Kara."

Clint drove to Clarksburg every day and worked ten to twelve hours a day, six days a week. He told me he felt okay, just not right. He still wasn't sleeping. His hips still ached on and off, but again, not too much. I tried to think positive thoughts, but it was hard to do that after everything he had gone through.

February 2009

I heard the garage door go up. "Mom," Clint yelled from the basement as he headed to the shower. "I'm all done. That job is finished. I made it through. I didn't always feel the best, but I made it through. And I didn't miss one day. Now, I need to find another job."

I was relieved, but I knew his story wasn't over. The pain wasn't over. I didn't say anything to Clint about my concerns. I just said what he needed me to say. "That's wonderful. You're amazing! You did the impossible."

March 2009

As usual, Clint had a job within two weeks of putting his name back out there. He was going to Huntington to work at a Marathon Oil refinery. It would be cold. He would be working on towers. It was dangerous work. He was excited.

"Mom, I'm out of here! I'll be back in a couple of weeks. It's not that far away. If I need Kara, I can be home in four and a half hours. It'll be okay." He was trying to calm me down. I guess he could tell by the look on my face that I was extremely worried.

I followed him out to the garage and stood by his truck as he drove away. I saw him looking at me in his rearview mirror. All I could do was hope for the best while silently fearing the worst.

Clint called me often from the job. The work was tough, and the wind was cold. It was breaking him down. The urinating issue never completely stopped. It just lessened. He still was not sleeping much. He took a Valium every once in a while, at night, to help.

While Clint was gone, almost without my noticing it, Garin and I started going on dates. Since Clint seemed to be getting better, I was able to relax and enjoy Garin's company again.

June 2009

I heard the garage door go up. "Mom," Clint called as he headed toward the shower. "The job's over. I have my layoff papers. I don't feel a hundred percent. I think I am going to take a month off and go see Kara again.

"They wanted me to go to Texas, but I don't think I can. I'm sad that I can't do it. I'm just not feeling up to it, and I really should stay close to Kara. I have to get back to the pelvic-floor therapy."

I sighed. I knew this would happen. Something I couldn't figure out was very wrong. Again, I searched for answers via the internet. Still, there was little information regarding heavy-metal poisoning and metal toxicity. I did run across some articles about over body burden. The term refers to a body's total accumulations of toxins.

Clint spent the next few months working with Kara. Because he focused on resting and taking care of himself, he felt better again.

As I recall, Garin and I went camping, not once but twice before the weather turned cold.

October 2009

I heard the garage door go up. "Mom!" Clint called excitedly. "I'm going back to work! It's close, less than ten minutes from the house. My welding buddies and I are going to design and build tanks in South Charleston. Just the three of us; it'll be fun."

"That sounds nice," I lied. I was worried out of my mind. That is what I did in those days: worry.

Clint and his friends had a good time doing the job. They had fun together. Clint had enough time to do his pelvic exercises, rest, and work. He was improving again. Perhaps he improved too much.

Eleven

Coming Home to Die (2010–2011)

February 2010

The winter was harsh and full of snow. Although Garin had stopped over and cleared a track for my car before he left for work, I was determined to shovel the rest of the driveway clear. Deep in my own thoughts, I hardly noticed Clint pull into the driveway.

"Mom!" he yelled from his truck. "We're going to New Orleans." I looked up from my snow pile in shock.

"I'm sorry. What?"

"I'm leaving as soon as I can pack my stuff. There's a company down there that just hired my buddy to work the refinery. He's taking me with him."

Crap, I thought, my nerves jangling. "How wonderful," I said supportively. "You'd better start packing. What do you need me to do?"

"Nothing! I just need to load my gang box and get my clothes packed. Then I'll be on the road again," he hollered. He was grinning ear to ear, so excited to be going back on the road again.

He had an eight-hour drive ahead of him. I was worried, but he had come a long way. I had to have hope. I had to find trust in his future.

A few minutes later, I followed Clint to his truck, snow shovel in hand, and waved goodbye. "Bye, Clint. I love you! Be safe. Make sure you call a lot."

Clint knew I was worried. He shot me a big Clint grin. "Mom," he said in a reassuring tone, "this is a good thing. I only have that urgent feeling of needing to pee occasionally now. My hips have stopped hurting most of the time. I'm not sick to my stomach anymore. I don't feel exactly right quite yet, but look at me. I'm getting there." He turned on his truck's engine, shot me another big grin that had been missing since 2005, and slowly pulled away. "I love you! See you soon!"

My cell phone rang a lot while Clint was in New Orleans. It was Mardi Gras, and he was having a blast. He sent me pictures of the parades. He was laughing. The old Clint was back.

Why did I worry? I asked myself. *Maybe Garin has been right all along, and everything really* is *all right.* But moms know. They are connected to the souls of their children. We just know!

Then Clint moved to Arkansas to work at another refinery. His buddies had moved on and taken other jobs in different states. Clint stayed with the company to which his friend had introduced him. He liked the work, and he was very good, doing the job.

It was extremely hot, and safety was the number-one priority. Clint had to wear a protective suit and respirator most of the time. He was not able to drink the amount of water that he needed to be drinking each day. Workers were not allowed to carry anything into the secured area. Explosions were a constant threat, so the job was highly regulated. It was an extremely long walk to the water source in the plant. Once again, he was doing tower work. This meant he was climbing stairs to the top with about twenty-five pounds of tools on his waist, turning the same direction every ten feet. The grinding on his hips and back was taking its toll on his already frail body.

"Mom," Clint said when I answered my phone a few weeks later. "My hip pain is coming back. It's bad. I don't want to give up and come home, but my bladder is starting to give me fits too."

I had been afraid this day would come. "Oh, Clint," I murmured.

"My back hurts, and I don't feel well. I'm coming home. I will stay as long as I can, but I'm going to need to come home soon."

My chest began pounding. My head began to throb. My brain was spinning as I said goodbye. I went into the bathroom and threw up.

The battle we had already fought was a walk in the park compared to the battle that was to follow.

April 2010

"Mom," Clint whispered in my ear. "I'm the last man on the job. Everyone else has been let go. The shutdown is almost over. As usual, I am the last man left. They want me to go to Texas. I'm not going to be able to do it. I have to come home. I think I'm coming home for good. This is *really* bad. I can't do this again. I am going down to Alabama to see Grams."

He thinks he is going to die! I realized with dismay. *He wants to see his grandma to say goodbye.*

He said the pain was moving around inside of him and growing in intensity by the hour. "I'm leaving tomorrow to visit with Grams. I'll be home in about ten days."

I told him to be careful and spend some time with his grandma without telling her how sick he really was. I urged him not to worry her.

"Come home, and I will figure this out," I told him. "It will be okay. I always figure things out. Have I ever not?" Nervously, I asked, "Are you sure this is a good decision? It's four hours south, and then you have to make it home. You know you are going to hurt more as the days pass."

"Mom, I have to spend some time with my grandma. What happens if this is the end? I think this might be the end. I cannot go through this again. What if my pelvic-floor disease is back? We have been trying since 2004 to find out what is wrong. I am out of doctors. You are out of rabbits to pull out of your hat. No more rabbits. I am done. There is nothing we can do since my doctors don't listen."

Clint came home as promised. Exhaustion etched dark circles under his eyes and deeply into his cheeks. His eyes looked dull, and his skin was yellow again. He was having trouble urinating. His hips would lock in place, and his elbows would lock in a bent position. He was hungry but couldn't eat. He wasn't sleeping more than a few moments at a stretch. Every symptom he had worked so hard to chase away was back—every single one. He had a rash all over his body, mostly on his back, chest, and neck. If he ate eggs, it got worse. This was a very important clue that I totally missed. Hindsight is twenty-twenty.

I knew we were missing something. He reminded me of a middle-aged woman going through menopause. I decided to take him to a hormone clinic.

His pain became so intense; he was constantly throwing up. Because of all the throwing up and his inability to eat, he was losing weight fast.

Every night, I heard him in the basement, hugging the toilet seat, vomiting all night long. He moaned in pain. He cried and cried. "Mom, I need to go see Kara. I need to know if I screwed up my pelvic-floor muscles again, climbing those 120-foot towers with all my gear on."

"Okay. That's a good idea. I'm looking for a hormone clinic so we can have your balances checked. Maybe that's why you can't sleep."

Clint went to see Kara within a few days of calling her. The good news was that his pelvic floor was perfect! There was no damage and no pelvic-floor disease. We had no need for a team of doctors, no need for a support group. The bad news was that she had no explanation for his condition.

The question remained, what was causing his pain? If the bladder issue was back, but the pelvic floor was healthy, did that mean that the pelvic-floor disease was just a symptom of something greater?

June 2010

Clint's pain was horrendous. He couldn't stop vomiting. His hips were completely locked up. Out of stupidity or desperation, we decided to go to the hospital OEMS (Office of Emergency Medical Services) emergency room. This had never worked in the past, but his pain was so intense, we felt we had no other option. We had been to almost every emergency room in Charleston with this pain. Having taken no time with such frivolities as hairstyling and makeup, I didn't look great, and Clint was screaming in pain.

We were labeled as codependent drug seekers. Clint kept saying not to give him narcotics, to try something else, anything else. The doctors and nurses were rude and assuming.

"They don't work," he explained. "I don't want pain pills. I just need something to knock me out for a few hours so I can sleep." The medical staff looked at him like he had three heads. They gave him an intravenous bag of something that was supposed to help with the pain and let him relax. It had no effect.

"Here is what we can do for you," the doctor said as we were being discharged. "We made an appointment for you at the indigent orthopedic clinic. They are backed up, so they can't get you in for two months. You'll have to wait."

I looked at Clint, and he stared back with a look of confusion and outrage. Clint had money, and he'd had a job until recently. He had insurance. He didn't need to go to a clinic for the needy or poor.

With Clint's medical history, a low-income clinic seemed to be a very poor choice. Rather than taking that advice, I decided to call Dr. Arens, an orthopedic doctor associated with CAMC, whose name I had found in the phone book. This doctor had very good reviews on the internet.

Very good reviews, I repeated to myself as I called for an appointment.

July–October 2010

"Come on. Let's go," I said. "Perhaps we should have been pushing harder on your hip pain issue instead of going the urologist route." We had followed the advice of urologists many times. It seemed like no doctor took Clint seriously. Everybody found it easier to label him neurotic, if not psychotic.

Clint could hardly walk. He was leaning on my shoulder as we entered Dr. Arens's office. Dr. Arens came into the room. He was a little guy who wore a goofy green tweed suit jacket and an awkwardly large bow tie. He was extremely short and seemed to have a defensive, angry personality. Normally, I like differently or oddly dressed people, but his body language seemed to tell me that he dressed that way for the wrong reason.

Oh dear, I thought as I watched him approach.

He asked Clint all the same questions again. The same ones everyone always asked us. Again, the new doctor was certain that Clint needed another x-ray. Then he needed an MRI. All of this caused more exposure to heavy metals.

Gadolinium poisoning is becoming a growing health problem. Researchers suspect it stays in the brain and causes both brain abnormalities and kidney damage.

In an article published in February 2017, the Lighthouse Project—an organization that "sheds light on the effects of retained gadolinium"—

released their comprehensive report of retained gadolinium in a patient with normal kidney function. It is their feelings that 1 percent of the injected gadolinium from each dose of contrast is retained in the body. Multiple contrast MRIs compound the level of toxicity (www.gadoliniumtoxicity.com).

Clint's medical records documented five years of urological problems. He was diagnosed with pelvic-floor dysfunction. Yet no doctor who saw Clint ever considered the added burden to his broken body when they ordered tests. When I asked questions, I was brushed aside as a uneducated, interfering mom. This visit was no different than the ones before. Dr. Arens talked down to me and Clint. I just cannot understand why.

"Can you help me out with this pain? I haven't slept in months," Clint asked.

"No," Dr. Arens said, squinting up at Clint. "I don't prescribe pain medication. If that's what you're looking for, you're in the wrong place. I can refer you to a pain-management doctor."

We left and scheduled the MRI. As in the past, after the MRI Clint's symptoms worsened. The inflammation in his body increased as his body fought to flush out the gadolinium. I stored that thought to ask Dr. Arens what he knew about gadolinium poisoning.

In two weeks, we returned to Dr. Arens for the test results, expecting a plan to repair the hips, whatever that meant. Clint leaned on me again as we walked into Dr. Arens's office. What happened next is so unbelievable I have to keep reminding myself I'm not making it up.

Clint looked like he was on death's doorstep. I was exhausted from working around the clock, so I'm sure I didn't look much better. I had a nine-month accounting project that kept me up until two thirty in the morning most nights. I was going to offices to work from seven thirty in the morning until six o'clock in the evening. Beyond that, I was taking care of my dying son all the time.

Had Garin not been stopping in to do some of the cooking, I probably wouldn't have eaten any more than Clint did. Mechanically, I went through the motions of eating and other mundane routines. The house became a danger zone of cobwebs and piles of unattended stuff. Laundry was washed but never put away. Repeatedly, I just selected an outfit from the dryer as I headed out the door, exhausted from the pressure of wearing so many hats.

Repeatedly, Clint stood at the foot of the bed, shaking in pain. When I whispered to him to go, my son would shuffle away.

I heard the garage door go up and down. Many times, Clint would be outside all night long, breathing deeply in an attempt to release endorphins to help the pain. He would walk the road to try to stretch out his hips and leg muscles because they were all cramped up. He would sit on the front step and stretch and cry in pain. I woke up nightly, hearing him crying on the basement floor and hearing the toilet flush ten to twenty times a night. We were in a living hell.

Then this clown of a doctor walked in and told us, "You have necrosis of the femoral heads. This is caused by steroid and alcohol abuse. I can't help you. You asked for this. I can refer you to someone else. He can cut off the top of your hips and replace them with metal ones. But remember: you made the choices, and you're going to have to live with the results."

I was shaking as Clint began to cry. We had reached another dead end down a dark, painful road. He was just another arrogant, mean-spirited doctor that refused to do his job. Crying, Clint pleaded, "I need help, Doctor. I'm dying. I can feel myself dying! There's something in me, eating me away from the inside. It's not going to stop unless you help me. Can't you even give me something to help me sleep? I don't drink. I have never taken steroids. I am sick. Can you please help me?"

"No." That word had been the simple answer handed to us many times, but it hurt to hear it again. "Goodbye. My nurse will arrange the appointment with the new orthopedic doctor." He briskly walked out the door and never returned. Clint grabbed hold of my shoulder, and we limped out to the front desk to make another appointment. We had to wait another six weeks for the new doctor's appointment. Dr. Arens never gave the respect or time for me to ask my question about the MRI and gadolinium toxicity. He never said goodbye. In mid-sentence, he turned his back to us and walked out the door.

Clint and I both cried all the way home. Clint stood in the driveway and watched me pull away. "I have to go to work," I told him. "I'll be home tonight. We'll figure something out then. I have bills to pay. Sorry; I wish I didn't, but I have to go."

I watched Clint turn toward the house and limp all the way inside. I drove to work on autopilot while my brain was someplace else.

Clint was so angry. He didn't drink. He never took steroids. Why was this happening? Why was everyone being so accusing and hateful?

While I was at work, Clint decided to drive one mile away and do a walk-in visit with the local Lighthouse Orthopedic Office. He just limped in and stood in front of the desk. The young girl at the desk knew Clint was about to pass out from pain. She took him back into their office and began to ask him questions. The nurse took his vitals, and no one there would let him leave. How strange! Dr. Arens threw him out, and Lighthouse wouldn't let him leave.

The next day at four in the afternoon, Clint had an appointment with Dr. Khanna. Did you catch that? Not six weeks. Not eight weeks. Less than twenty-four hours later!

I went along because Clint could hardly walk. He couldn't sit or lie down.

Clint was sent back for his first set of x-rays with Dr. Khanna. Dr. Khanna used the first set to look for problems. He sent Clint back for more x-rays. No one in the entire practice had ever seen anything like this. They just kept taking more images with the hips in different positions. The arthritis was so bad they could not figure out how he was even walking.

Dr. Khanna put the x-rays on the back-lit x-ray board again. More people in the office came to look. Clint was sent back for more. Dr. Khanna and the medical staff looked at all the x-rays. And Clint and I were looking at each other, watching all of this through the open patient room door, wondering and waiting.

Finally, Dr. Khanna came in, sat in front of us, and began. "Clint, you have a lot going on. It's a mess. You need to see Dr. Savvin on his first available appointment. West Virginia Power is playing ball out of town. He is their team doctor—he travels with them—but he will be back on August 21. I know that he will fit you in as soon as he looks at your x-rays."

Clint and I were stumped. My chest tightened, and my head felt like it was spinning off my neck. I felt like I might throw up. Clint's eyes were wide, the size of half dollars.

"There are issues, serious issues," Dr. Khanna explained. "But Dr. Savvin can help you. You will have to wait eleven days."

While we waited for the August 21 appointment, Lighthouse gave Clint relief from his pain with steroid injections. The swelling had to be shut down before Dr. Savvin could do anything surgically. For the first time in four years, the pain in Clint's hips was temporarily stopped.

Dr. Savvin worked out of a Charleston office on the other side of town from our home. The ride was painful for Clint to endure. As I drove, we practiced the dos and don'ts of what to say to doctors. Clint kept coaching me not to bring up his past year's medical mystery. He kept repeating that the hip pain was totally separate from the urinary and other medical conditions that still had not been correctly diagnosed. We did a little role-playing, and I was ready for another performance. It just frustrated me that a patient had to hold back the truth in order to get the medical treatments he needed. Clint limped in while I parked the car. We came prepared.

What an amazing place, I thought as I walked into the waiting room.

Clint and I felt that we were in the right place for his hip problem. As a sports medicine facility, it was all about rebuilding to ultimately get back into the game. With its bright, open lobby and athletic-type furniture, it was the antithesis of an "end of the road; let's give up" kind of place like we had been visiting. *Promising,* I thought. We both knew it was not the answer to his medical problem with the body breakdown—but at least he finally had someone who said yes. "Yes, we understand you have severe hip pain, and we can fix it!"

Dr. Savvin came into the patient room with a big smile on his face and introduced himself. After the introductions, he got down to business. "I've looked at all of your x-rays, and you're in a real mess. How'd you do this to yourself?"

Clint told his story. He talked about dirt-bike riding and described some crashes. Then he described his job and explained how he would climb 120-foot towers with heavy tool belts. Clint and I had learned: give the Western-licensed doctor what he wanted. Give him an acceptable reason why you were sick. Don't go off the straight-and-narrow path. Comply with required insurance code diagnoses, or get no help.

If you sway, you'll be sent away! The words jingled in my mind as we sat with Dr. Savvin that day.

"You have the hips of a fifty-eight-year-old," Dr. Savvin explained, surprised and concerned about Clint's condition. "I have never seen anything like this before. You must be one tough guy. Your labrum has been shredded off your left hip. How'd you do that? I wonder. Have you been playing soccer, football, baseball?" Clint shook his head. "Like I said, I've never ever seen this. I'm surprised you're still walking with a torn labrum. Athletes roll around on the ground when they have this injury. They get carried off the field, crying like babies. You've been working? Still? Climbing towers?" he asked. Clint nodded. "This didn't just happen in the past few weeks. This has been this way for at least a few months. You have several bone spurs that shred your labrums. I'm going to schedule surgery for you in ten days. I would do it tomorrow if I wasn't leaving town with the Power."

Clint and I exchanged a look, jointly confused over what had just happened, and then nodded agreement to the surgery. Three weeks ago, Dr. Arens had accused us of being drug seekers and had told Clint he deserved this pain.

"Thank you. Thank you so much," Clint said with immense gratitude. "No one else would listen to me. You can see I'm a mess. I really need to go back to work. I'm a pipe fitter, so I need my hips to work."

"You belong here," Dr. Savvin said with a grin. "I'm going to take care of you. I'll remove all the osteoarthritis and try to save the labrum. I'll pop those bone spurs right off. I'll know more of what I can do to help you once I'm in there, but I promise you I'll do everything I can to get you back into fighting shape. I'd like to at least get you back to 90 percent functionality. I can't figure out how this happened to you." Dr. Savvin shook his head with surprise at Clint's state as he closed the examination room door. He left us stunned.

Both of Clint's hips were locked up with osteoarthritis. His left was worse than his right. The labrum on the right was still intact, so Dr. Savvin decided that the left had to be worked on first. Because the right could not be fixed at the same time, Clint couldn't start total rehabilitation. Clint was scheduled to have surgery on his left hip ten days later, on August 31. Then he'd have almost twelve weeks to rehab before his doctor would address the right hip.

The surgery on his left hip was a success. Dr. Savvin was able to save the labrum, as he had hoped. I watched the entire operation from the observation room. Other medical professionals who worked with Dr. Savvin were in the room with me. They commented that this was the toughest surgery they'd ever seen. I guess that's why Dr. Savvin asked them to watch. He knew Clint's procedure was going to be one of his best operating-room performances. Everyone in the surgical room wore rain gear—there was water everywhere, perhaps because it was required to cool the equipment. The leg they were working on was on the other side, so I couldn't see everything directly. I could watch on the TV on the wall or through the window where they were working in the OR. But there was a constant rush of water behind Clint's hip, and the water would shoot up once in a while. The raincoats everyone wore were wet. The floor had about two inches of water on it by the time they were finished.

Dr. Savvin worked through a tiny incision in Clint's thigh. He used what I would call a blowtorch to melt the labrum flat. It appeared to be crumpled and knotted up. It looked like a thick milk carton looks after being run over by a car. While he was using the blowtorch, Clint's leg looked like it caught fire but was quickly put out.

Dr. Savvin shot a pop rivet into Clint's hip bone, and then attached a string that looked like dental floss onto that rivet. He flattened the labrum onto the hip bone and tied it down with the floss. In his notes, Dr. Savvin noted he did that twice, just to be sure it stayed put. *Thank you, Dr. Savvin.*

When all the white fuzz that surrounded Clint's hip was removed and the floss was tied down, they closed up Clint. I was sitting on a chair, watching through a large window, afraid to move. Dr. Savvin came to the window, and I will never forget this: Peering at me, he lifted his right arm and put the back of his wrist to his forehead. He pulled his hand away as he mouthed, *"Phew!"*

I smiled at the notion—and trust me, I felt the same way. He gave me a thumbs-up, "we did it" sign and walked away. Everyone in the room clapped.

I must express my total appreciation for Lighthouse at this point. Everywhere I had been with Clint, we had been treated poorly, disrespected, and unfairly suspected. Doctors had talked down to me like I was stupid. Up to this point, that had *never* happened at Lighthouse.

Dr. Savvin was done with one procedure, and he had saved the labrum and the left hip. Clint and I knew that metal hip replacements wouldn't be a good thing. Around that time, lawsuits were starting regarding the hip replacements that had caused the disease called *metallosis*.

Metallosis is a putative medical condition involving deposition and buildup of metal debris in the soft tissues of the body. The symptoms were very similar to Clint's. With these new developments, people were beginning to discuss heavy-metal toxicity on the internet.

Presumably, Dr. Savvin, like the other doctors, did not want to hear about heavy-metal exposure, so I kept quiet about it. Clint needed these surgeries, and he needed them immediately. This doctor was our only hope.

October 2010

While Clint was still on crutches from his surgery, he and I went to BioIdentity in downtown Charleston to see a specialist who treated hormone imbalances.

BioIdentity did a lot of tests, none of which were covered by insurance. The bill was about $1,500. *Surely,* I thought, *we'll find out something!*

"Come on, Clint," I said. "Your appointment with Bio-Identity is in thirty minutes. I can't wait to hear the results of the tests."

Three weeks had elapsed since Clint's surgery. He was going to therapy twice a week and doing therapeutic exercises twice every day. In extreme pain from the surgery, while still suffering with heavy-metal poisoning, he had yellowish skin and bags under his eyes, announcing that he hadn't slept well in months. His muscles were gone. He looked like a shambling member of the walking dead.

Soon, Clint and I were sitting across from the doctor in anticipation of the results.

"I have never seen tests results like this," the doctor started. We were nervous. We'd heard that before. "I'll be honest; I don't understand what's going on. I will have to have my associate who designed the tests read them and let me know what to do. In the meanwhile, I want you to start taking some supplements and change your diet.

"Your hormones are just gone. It seems like your adrenal glands have shut down. You don't have any testosterone, vitamin D, or HDL—good cholesterol. And your liver is in failure! I have no idea why this is happening. I have never ever seen anything like this before. Your trace minerals are missing. Some are too high, some are too low, and others are just gone. The really weird one is the high amount of calcium that's in your blood." She must have seen our nervousness at the overload of information. "But don't worry! Give me six months, and you will feel better."

Oh my God, how many times will I hear this? I wondered. That bit of information and the supplement purchase cost me about two thousand dollars.

Clint and I went back every month with little to no change. "This takes time," the doctor explained. "You have to give your body time to heal. Something happened to you, and it will take months to fix. I am going to add a few more supplements for you to take." The monthly cost for this service and supplements was $450.

"Did you get a chance to review Clint's test with the other doctors?" I asked. Stumbling over her words, she mentioned something about having to follow up on that. I wanted to say something to make her understand this was not satisfactory. But I had so many other things to worry about, I dropped it. In future years, I think I finally understood why my questions were never answered.

Clint did have some days that weren't so bad—again. He was working day and night to rehabilitate his left hip in preparation for surgery on the right. He couldn't exercise at full force until after the right hip surgery was completed, but he was determined to build enough strength to support his entire body in preparation for the next surgery, when he would not be permitted to put any weight on the right hip.

He was still losing weight, and his skin had a definite yellow cast. Skin rashes erupted with increasing frequency, and the bladder issue had not gone away. He continued daily to follow the protocol for keeping his pelvic floor strong.

I am 100 percent sure that Clint's illness was due to heavy-metal exposure. Everywhere I've gone and asked questions, I have been told that it's impossible. "Metals don't stay in the body. He must be depressed. Take him to a pain-management clinic, and get him some help."

None of it made sense. Where did this all come from? Where did it start? He was working in 2004. He had pushed through all the tough days of finding himself and then proving to people that he was good at his trade. Why now? Why didn't the depression and anxiety happen when he was twenty-one and had nothing to offer toward his future? The depression theory had no basis in fact.

Yet let's stop a minute and consider this: Lawsuits are hitting the news. Metallosis is the putative medical condition involving deposition and buildup of metal debris in the soft tissues of the body. Why can people who've had the misfortune of needing metal hip replacements be allowed to name their disease with a cause, other than depression or anxiety? Let me get this straight: Workers who are daily exposed to heavy-metal ions on the job site cannot get overburdened, but people who have daily exposure to heavy-metal ions from hip implants demonstrably do? What is the difference? Perhaps it's the same reason that OHSA and NIOSH don't care about sick workers unless it's acute or a huge accident. Perhaps it's nothing more complicated or mysterious than the adage "Follow the money."

Clint kept working out. He never quit. He just kept going.

December 2010

"Come on, Clint. Get up," I whispered into Clint's room. At four thirty in the morning, it was still dark outside. "Surgery is in three hours." It was time to fix the right hip. Clint had done the seemingly impossible. Somehow, he had sufficiently strengthened the left hip for Dr. Savvin to agree to do the right hip on schedule. Dr. Savvin was once again in total shock when Clint came in for his evaluation appointment to see if the left hip was strong enough to operate on the right. Post-hip surgery rehabilitation typically requires two years of therapy. Clint's entire body was dying, yet he did it.

Thankfully, the surgery was not as long or difficult as the last. That's not saying much, considering the last surgery took twice as long as expected. Dr. Savvin once again did a fabulous job. He was professional and kind. He's a tough guy, proving if you do the work, he does too.

By Christmas, Clint was seriously rebuilding his hip strength. His bladder problem was still an issue, and he felt like crap in general. He continued going to physical therapy two times a week and working out at home twice a day. Things were looking up, at least in regard to his hips.

Twelve

Black Hats and White Hats (2011–2012)

February 2011

Dr. Savvin checked in on Clint occasionally when he was working out and always said he was doing a great job. Clint never stopped—until February, when suddenly the hip pain returned.

The pain was a little different this time. It started in the center of his hips and ran down his buttocks, through his groin, and extended down his legs. Back pain returned as well.

Clint tried to tell them his pain was back, but Dr. Savvin didn't want to hear it. His personal assistant became impatient and guarded with Clint. After a while, she became downright mean. One day, while Clint was trying to explain what he thought was wrong, she called him a pussy.

"I told you this would be the worst sporting event of your life," Dr.

Savvin lectured Clint. "I told you this was not going to be easy. Get back in the game! You need to keep going to get better. You can't turn back." He sounded like an angry football coach.

Where had this come from? What was going on? Clint tried to continue with his therapy. But the pain wasn't subsiding. Clint knew Dr. Savvin simply could not understand what was wrong with him.

"Clint, I found a new therapy center for you to go to," I said. "It's only five minutes from the house, and they incorporate other pain-relieving therapies as well. I think this will be better than creating more pain at Lighthouse."

The new therapy center discovered that Clint had a torn gluteus maximus, most likely caused by the extreme physical therapy. They taped Clint's butt cheek and thigh to promote healing and stop the pain. The pain subsided a little but did not go away.

I contacted an occupational rehabilitation center on Wildbend Road. Clint went there in April.

A fresh MRI showed that Clint had necrosis, a form of cell injury that results in the premature death of cells in living tissue by autolysis. Necrosis is caused by factors external to the cell or tissue—such as infection, toxins, or trauma—that result in the unregulated digestion of cell components. In contrast, apoptosis is a naturally occurring, programmed, and targeted cause of cellular death. While apoptosis often provides beneficial effects to the organism, necrosis is almost always detrimental and can be fatal.

In my research on avascular necrosis, I looked for the cause and what could be done to slow its progression. I found a wealth of information. Also called osteonecrosis, avascular necrosis can lead to tiny breaks in the bone and the bone's eventual collapse. Necrosis, which is caused by the lack of oxygen in red blood cells, could be caused by arsenic, I discovered.

I thought about this. *How can we get oxygen into his blood?* I researched hyperbaric oxygen chambers. Hyperbaric means pertaining to a gas at greater pressure than normal. With a chamber, Clint could have hyperbaric oxygen therapy (HBOT), a medical treatment that enhances the body's natural healing process by inhalation of 100 percent oxygen in a total body chamber, where atmospheric pressure is increased and controlled.

Bingo-bango! We need one of those now, I thought. I looked at different models, the location from which the chamber would ship, and how long it would take to have it at my house. For $6,500, I could have a home hyperbaric oxygen chamber delivered in less than two weeks.

I called several doctor offices in Charleston, as well as the area hospitals, to see if Clint could come into their offices for hyperbaric treatments. The cost was way more than just purchasing our own. If this treatment was going to have any effect on the necrosis, he would need to go into the chamber twice a day, every day of the week. Clint had to have his own chamber for this to work.

I knew Clint was running out of time, and I had to stop the cellular death in those hips. Money, costs, bills? By then, it was too late to care. I jumped through all the hoops to have the chamber shipped to West Virginia. I overcame the issues with owning one. I was in this to save my son, and *no* wasn't an answer I was willing to consider. I am a warrior and my great-aunt was giving me her strength as well. I was not giving up.

The chamber arrived in ten days. Clint was in it two times a day. Still sleeping very little, he would get up at five in the morning and climb straight into the chamber. I sat with him as it came to pressure, and then I jumped into the shower to get ready for work. Clint had the remote inside with him and could adjust the pressure as needed. I would get everything ready for my day while he was in the chamber. At six thirty he would come out, and I would leave for work. His breakfast was made, his lunch was inside the cooler next to his chair, and dinner was planned.

May 2011

"Clint, get ready. We have to go see Dr. Khanna." The effort to try to save Clint's hips had begun again. We went back to Lighthouse Orthopedics.

Dr. Khanna walked into the patient room and greeted us.

No one was as friendly as they were in August 2010. I was trying to figure out what game they were playing. *Should I be playing? How?* I wondered.

Dr. Khanna started to talk at a very hesitant pace, as if he was thinking in between each statement. "You have necrosis." Pause. "Sometimes this just happens." Pause. "Sometimes, bones just die." Pause. "Sometimes it's alcohol-related, and sometimes it's a result of steroid abuse." Pause. "In your case, I have no idea." Pause. "The cause doesn't matter. What does matter is the timing." Pause. "There is a small window, and then it will be too late. Your hip bones are dying, and we need to save them. So let's get started."

I looked over at Clint; he had tears in his eyes. I wanted to cry too. Then I asked the forbidden question. "I've been doing some research, and there's another cause. It's called metal poisoning. You might have heard—it's called over body burden. It's all over the internet. Information wasn't there when this all started, but it's there now. What do you think? Could it be that?"

Dr. Khanna fidgeted in his chair and restacked the papers he was holding. He was thinking. He looked up at me, nervousness engulfing his features.

Clint shot me a look with fire shooting out of his eyes. I didn't stay the course. I went to the forbidden land of heavy-metal poisoning. I could see in his face that he was scared to death that we were about to be kicked out.

"I've never heard of that," Dr. Khanna said.

For heaven's sake, I thought, *you do metal hip replacements. You must know!*

Of course, he knows, I thought. *If he said yes, I would have a medical doctor to subpoena. His loss of billable surgical time while he sat in court was not worth saving Clint's life.*

"That's really not my area. Either way, the hips have to have decompression procedures now. Let's set you up for May 24. All set? Good. I'll see you then." He left the room quickly, without waiting for our response.

Once again, Clint's back was up against the wall. He had no choice. He had to move ahead with a very dangerous surgical procedure. He was still dying from the inside out. The hips were proof of that.

Dr. Khanna's assistant came in and set up everything. Clint was going to have another invasive, destructive surgery, fewer than seven months from the others. This was unheard of.

As we headed for the car, Clint let me have it. "Mom, how could you do that? How could you break our sacred agreement? How? What happens if he calls and says he cannot see me anymore? What happens if I get kicked out of another medical practice? I can't believe you did this!"

I was so mad with myself. Clint was right. I didn't follow proper doctor protocol. I failed. I wanted to cry. "Please God, please let this scheduled decompression procedure happen."

Clint was dying from the inside out, as he had been saying since 2005. This was proven. Without a doubt, it was proven with the necrosis diagnosis. Yet not one doctor would listen to him. Again, I ask why?

Painful days came and went. My nights were confusing. *Did I sleep?* I wondered repeatedly, for I woke exhausted every morning. My chest felt tight, and my head was in a constant state of fog. It felt like I had spent the night working out, as every muscle in my body ached.

After getting Clint set up in the chamber, I headed for the shower. I wished the water could wash all of this misery from my war-torn body.

Wanting to run away from everything, I gave myself the usual pep talk. *It's okay. It's okay. All I need is a cup of coffee with lots of cream and sugar to get me going.*

"Clint, it's time to go," I called. "It's four thirty. Surgery is in three hours." Dr. Khanna was doing the first hip decompression that morning. The clock was ticking; Clint was on cellular death's doorstep.

In my understanding, hip decompression is this: The hip has one blood supply to the femoral head. That red blood supply has to be rich in oxygen. The oxygen and red blood cells' job is to keep the white blood cells purging. The red blood cells collect the dead white cells and dump them off in the lymph nodes. If the white blood cells build up inside the hip's head, the hip becomes weak and collapses. A deformity of the ball at the top of the femur is called cam impingement. When this happens, the usual solution is to replace the hips with metal ones.

But metal hips were not an option. Clint couldn't have metal hips! I knew metal implants leach heavy metals, and that would kill him for sure. As I've previously mentioned, by this time there was much information on the internet about metal hip replacements causing a new disease called metallosis. Lawsuits were all over the news, and DuPuy hips were being recalled. They were in big trouble.

Having been created in 2007, this decompression surgery had not been done for long. The doctor told us that Clint had a 75 percent chance that the decompression would work for three years. After that, there were no success rate records, no records at all.

I drove Clint to Ashton Center to a recently built hospital and dropped him off at the door so he wouldn't have to walk from the parking lot. A few minutes later, I met him inside. *This is getting very old,* I thought. Then: *I am getting very old!*

Dr. Khanna came in. "Are you ready?"

What could we say? No, Clint's scared shitless, and so am I? We couldn't say that. So we just nodded our heads.

As I had during one of our previous appointments, I asked, "Is there any way that you can test the bones chips when you drill that hole through his femur bone? I want to know what metals are in him."

Dr. Khanna gave me a stern look and was cautious with his words. "No one has ever asked me that before. I don't think the hospital has the capability to do that."

I wanted to argue but didn't. *What do you mean no one has ever asked you this before? I did, a couple of weeks ago.* But I knew this is not the time to start any problems. He was about to take total control of Clint's future. I needed him as a friend, not an enemy.

"Well, then, can I have the bone chips so I can send them to a lab myself?" I asked. Oh my, that was not a good question.

He fumbled with his paperwork and looked at the floor. "Once those bone chips are removed from Clint they become property of the hospital. Hospital policy is not to allow anyone to take their body parts home," he said simply. That was that. It was settled. He left the room without looking at me.

The procedure seemed to go on and on. I paced. What else could I do? I thought Clint might die on the table. I was not at all sure I'd see him alive again. I sat and watched the computer screen that kept track of the patient's progress.

Dr. Khanna took a drill and bored into Clint's femur bone about four inches down his leg. I didn't get to watch this procedure, so I can only guess that it was not a construction heavy-duty concrete drill. That's what I imagined. Judging from the condition Clint was in after it was finished, I sometimes wonder. Dr. Khanna drilled through the center of the bone until he reached the cam impingement. Then he worked to remove the dead, compacted white blood cells that had accumulated in the top of Clint's leg. After that, Dr. Khanna packed the head with a calcium graft that included growth hormones.

I wasn't given the transcript of the surgery until I demanded a copy, months later. When I read that the bone chips had been gathered and sent to the pathology laboratory, I became very suspicious. Why couldn't they tell me what I wanted to know? What right did they have to send those bone samples to a lab without Clint's permission? What was I not being told? Why were there so many secrets? Why couldn't I have the chips checked for arsenic or lead? I wanted to know. Georgia Poison Control told me I *needed* to know. I could smell a rat.

Was the process a success? Only time would tell. Clint couldn't put any weight on his leg. His femur bone had a hole drilled into it. He couldn't step down and was back on crutches. We went home to wait and see. I became a postoperative nurse with absolutely no training. I was given this responsibility by default, yet I was not given any respect or even courtesy by the medical world when I asked questions.

I did more research. I wanted to figure out what Dr. Khanna knew that I didn't. Why had Lighthouse become so careful with their words? Why had their attitude become cold and detached toward a patient they once seemed to care for and praise? Something didn't seem right.

Information on the internet suggested a reason for necrosis that Dr. Khanna had failed to mention. Necrosis can be caused by a serious injury to the hip. It can be caused by a dislocated hip injury.

Dr. Savvin had to dislocate Clint's hips when he did the arthroscopy procedures last year. Does Lighthouse fear I am going to sue them? Does Lighthouse think they caused Clint's necrosis? I wondered with dismay. *Yes, I think they must. What a shame. Or do they suspect heavy metal toxicity and are not legally allowed to say?*

June 2011

Clint still didn't sleep much. His back hurt. He couldn't keep down much food. His ears bled. He constantly felt like he had to urinate. His eye kept getting a film growth on it that Dr. Schneider (who had done LASIK surgery on Clint when Clint was nineteen) could not explain.

I worried that Clint wouldn't even make it to the next surgery. And if he did, would he live through it? I desperately wanted it to end. Clint was dying to make it end.

He survived what I tried to tell myself was an accidental overdose. But I was coming to the point of total understanding if his intent had been focused.

The second time Clint was told he had avascular necrosis (AVN), I listened really well. And when I got home, I researched, like a crack addict looking for a fix, until I found the following: "AVN can be caused by steroids or alcohol abuse. It can also and it is more likely to be caused by heavy metals in our environment."

People come in contact with chemicals all day long. Most of the time, the liver is strong enough to clean them out. If a person has come in contact with too many metals, and the liver can't do its job, the heavy metals get trapped in the body. Soon after, symptoms like Clint's will appear.

Clint had a disease that led me to heavy metals, specifically arsenic and sulfuric acid. In later years, as more information became available on the internet, barium was also listed as a cause.

"Get on the phone and call all the guys who worked at ULTRA. I know there is something we missed," I told Clint. The warrior in me was screaming as the real battle was about to begin.

I mentally put on my suit of armor in anticipation of the next exhausting battle.

Clint called around—and the results were scary. Men in their mid-thirties had died of prostate cancer. Another friend in his thirties died from a heart issue while riding a motorcycle. Another man had the *exact* symptoms Clint was experiencing, and he told a parallel version of Clint's story, word for word, on the phone. I panicked.

We knew that the ULTRA plant in Pennsylvania had shut down and was in the middle of a multiple-year cleanup effort. Posing as an ULTRA employee, Clint called his old boss from ULTRA. The supervisor quickly became upset when Clint began to describe his symptoms since he left in 2004. He told Clint to call the Dallas office.

"They should be able to help you," the supervisor advised. "ULTRA takes care of their people." But what exactly did that mean?

Clint called Dallas and talked with several people there.

"Yes, it sounds like arsenic poisoning," they said. "When did you work in Pennsylvania? How long? What did you do for us?" Clint answered their questions without divulging he had been a subcontractor. They told him to get in touch with an ULTRA representative who was still in Pennsylvania. They promised they were going to help.

An hour later, Clint called the Pennsylvania representative. "I don't see your name on my employee listing on the computer. Are you sure you were an employee?"

"Why does that matter? I was there and worked for your company," Clint argued.

"It matters a lot. You need to go to the company that put you here to work. ULTRA can't help you if you weren't our employee. If you were a subcontractor, we're not legally responsible for your current condition. You need to contact *your* employer and work this out with them. Don't call back here," the man said.

Clint called Century Construction and told them about his health issues since leaving ULTRA. They told him that it happened "too long ago." They hadn't heard of anyone else getting sick. Like ULTRA, they chose to deny any knowledge or responsibility, stating there was no way Clint could prove any of this.

That didn't stop Clint. He called and called and called. He had a lot of anger to work out. What we had suspected all these years was true. ULTRA had known what they were doing.

My mind was spinning. I had a lot to do and very little time to get it done. I told Clint to think of his connections. When had he really begun to feel badly? Who could he call? What doors could we bang on for ideas? We needed help!

Clint called NIOSH (the National Institute for Occupational Safety and Health) and OSHA (the Occupational Safety and Health Administration). As part of the CDC (Centers for Disease Control), NIOSH is responsible for conducting research and making recommendations for the prevention of work-related illnesses and injuries. OSHA is the main federal agency charged with the enforcement of safety and health legislation.

Surprisingly, this turned out to be another waste of time.

"Did you call NIOSH or OSHA? Can they help us figure out where to go to get these metals removed?" I asked.

Clint said that neither NIOSH nor OSHA would talk to him. Needing to see for myself, I also called them.

"If it isn't acute poisoning, we don't care. We can't do anything about the past," a representative at NIOSH told me. I asked what they recommended for a person like Clint. They denied there was such a thing as chronic poisoning. NIOSH and OSHA support their employment by collecting money from violators. These were government employees who worked for and were paid by the government. Their job security was keeping their employer safe while supporting the accounts receivable department that supported their payroll department. Fines and penalties could be issued only in an accidental emergency situation. Blame and accountability was easy to prove; violations were recorded, and the responsible company paid whatever was assessed. Because there was no way to deny it didn't happen, the offender paid the fine. However, the injured worker paid the price for the rest of his or her life.

Government agencies work for the government, not for the US citizens who pay them. They do as the government tells them. I contend they are part of the cover-ups. If you doubt this, you might research Monsanto and

GMOs (genetically modified organisms). "Over the past decades, at least seven high ranking employees in the FDA at one time, were employed with Monsanto" (http://ivn.us/2013/02/11/the-revolving-door-fda-and-the-monsanto-company).

Follow the money.

Clint called West Virginia's Poison Center (WVPC) to ask for help, while I called the one in Georgia. Once again, Georgia was a waste of my time. As they had told me in 2007, I had to know the exact chemical or metal for which I was looking before they could help. WVPC told Clint to go to the CAMC (Charleston Area Medical Center) emergency room and get admitted to their toxicology department.

Reader, I'm glad that you've stuck with me through all that pain. Finally, I get to tell what I want and need to share!

The next morning, Friday, June 10, was rainy and dark, an ugly day outside. Clint was still on crutches and non-weight-bearing restrictions when we loaded into the car to head down to the CAMC emergency room.

I'd been trying for months to get an appointment with a toxicologist in Charleston. No toxicologist would take a person claiming to have had exposure more than seven years ago. Every single one of them said that it couldn't be arsenic poison. If it was, he would already be dead. No one would have lived through what I told them Clint did that day at ULTRA, all those years ago.

"It's illegal to have someone work in a closed environment like that. He'd have been terribly sick when he finished. He wouldn't have made it. It must not have happened. We can't see your son," they'd tell me.

Why are we going to the emergency room? I thought. *This is not an emergency. They're going to throw us out.* I kept my thoughts to myself. I looked over at Clint; he was so skinny. All of his muscles were completely gone. He was exhausted, yellow, and still in terrible pain. I was watching my son die. *I can't stop this train. What am I going to do?*

"Do you have insurance?" the young girl at the intake desk asked us.

That is always how it starts: insurance.

"Yes," Clint said and handed her his card.

Yes, he does. I pay for it, and most of the time, it's useless, I thought. *The doctors we see now don't take insurance. The doctors that do are useless.* With the exception of Lighthouse, they required insurance. However, I found out that the second osteoarthritis operation was declined by Clint's insurance company. Dr. Savvin did it anyway. He absorbed the cost. He knew it had to be done. Lighthouse never told me.

In 2004, until he left for Johns Hopkins Hospital, Clint was self-insured with WV Mutual. Two weeks before he was scheduled to leave for the clinic, WV Mutual canceled his policy. They had raised his rate to more than five hundred dollars a month, seeming to hope that he would drop them. We knew that he would never get insurance again with pelvic-floor disease and all the other misdiagnosed illnesses on his record, so I paid the ridiculous premiums. As it was, he was lucky. When WV Mutual canceled his policy, Clint's company allowed him to join theirs. Preexisting conditions are not a problem with group coverage. Self-payers are punished. So hard to believe, as we carry all the cost.

When he lost his job in 2007, he was eligible for coverage under COBRA (the Consolidated Omnibus Budget Reconciliation Act). We used no insurance while he was on the COBRA plan, so when it ended, there were no medical issues on his record. He was able to buy his own policy through Humana.

Humana has been great. Rates go up. But how much of this is Humana's greed, profit-producing hospitals, selfish doctors, or our own government?

"Mom!" Clint knocked me from my thoughts. We went from one waiting room to another. We arrived at 8:30; at 11:00 we were still waiting. On this trip, we entered the emergency room for a nonemergency visit, and they kept saying, "Why are you here? What do you want from us? This happened in 2004? Do you want pain medication?" Here we went again, with medical professionals assuming we wanted pain medication.

"No!" Clint answered in frustration. "They don't work for me. I have a new prescription from my last surgery, and I didn't even get it filled. I don't take them. What don't you understand?"

"What do you need? Why are you here?" they asked him again.

"I need someone to look over my medical history. The West Virginia Poison Center asked that you call them when I get here. They want to talk to you about my situation," Clint explained for perhaps the third time.

Something's wrong with these people, I could see them thinking. It was like there was a group thought bubble above their heads.

Clint was not given a private cubicle room. He was given a bed right outside the nurse's station. The emergency room coordinating physician came over to see us. I was sitting on a metal folding chair next to Clint, who sat, uncomfortably, waiting in the hospital bed. The entire emergency room staff went running by us all day long. The tiny Asian ER director possessed an extraordinarily kind face. As she listened to Clint's story, I could see the wheels spinning in her brain. She leaned back against a column and listened intently. She asked Clint for the contact at the WVPC and disappeared.

Clint and I waited for hours. We just sat there waiting as the emergency room activities overwhelmed us. Waiting. *But waiting for what?* I wondered. We could see the doctor on the phone. We watched her scanning the computer screen and furiously writing notes.

Finally, she and her associates came back to talk with us, her face scribbled with worry and sorrow. I'll never forget her words. "Yes, I can diagnose you with arsenic poisoning. I've been reviewing your medical records for three hours. You weren't sick before 2004, not even a cold. There's nothing in your history except accidents. Everything I've looked at points to arsenic.

"Unfortunately, there's nothing that can be done. Once it's in, it's in. It never comes out. You're going to die a slow and painful death."

Smackdown; it felt like the bedpan just hit me in the face.

My eyes met Clint's. Oh, dear Lord! This was what we had wanted to hear, that he had arsenic poisoning. *But he's going to die a slow and painful death? How long is that going to take? Aren't we already there?*

"Clint has been deathly sick since 2004," I explained to her. "I work fifty-five hours a week to pay his bills. I get up at four thirty every morning, fix his food for the day, and pack it in a cooler. I take a shower, say goodbye, and don't return until after six thirty. I'm exhausted, and Clint is home alone. I need help. We need help. Can we apply for hospice? If he's going to die, we should be able to get hospice. Right?"

She looked at me like I was a character from *The Exorcist*, wearing a bedpan.

"No, I'm so sorry. This diagnosis doesn't fit the criteria for hospice care. There isn't a code for death by arsenic."

My chest ached, and I clasped my hands together tightly in an attempt to hide their trembling. Feeling on the verge of a full-blown panic attack, I strove to formulate a fresh idea.

Clint sat there without moving. It was eerily as if he wasn't even in the room.

The doctor excused herself to get the discharge paperwork started. I stayed with Clint and tried to soothe him as he erupted in distress. "It's over. This has to stop!" he cried. "I'm just going to go home and find a way to kill myself!"

After I got him relatively calm, I needed to go outside to make phone calls regarding work that I had failed to show up for that day.

When I came back ten minutes later, Clint was sitting on the gurney, telling me to hurry up. "Where have you been?" he asked, though surely he had heard me when I had told him where I was going. "The doctor over there"—he nodded his head to the right—"came back while you were gone. Listen to me! You know my brain doesn't retain anything anymore, so I have to say this fast. She came over when no one else was nearby. She said, 'I am a Western-trained and licensed physician. There are certain thought processes here regarding metal toxicity. I will only say this one time, and I will deny ever saying it to you, so don't repeat it in here. You need to get out of the Western medical world. Run! Run as fast as you can. They're going to kill you. Arsenic can come out of your system, but you're going to need to an Eastern-trained doctor.'"

As Clint repeated the doctor's words, I realized what had been happening since 2004. Clint had been caught in the middle of a medical cover-up. Every doctor we went to refused to talk about heavy-metal poisoning. And if I pushed too hard, we were asked to leave and to never come back. If I pushed too hard, Clint and I were labeled mentally defective and sent on our way.

The bottom line was this: She couldn't open the doors to the toxicology department in the hospital. She had said the same thing we had already heard: "Only acute cases are allowed in there." If anyone suspected metal poisoning as a chronic condition, apparently, the patient was left to die!

Clint received his discharge papers, a prescription for Percocet, and a plastic jug in which to collect urine to send to a laboratory for testing. No one at the hospital could tell us how to do the test or where to send it. They just gave us the jug. "Call the local Lab Core group; they can tell you what to do."

Clint held up the prescription for the narcotics. "When will doctors listen to me? I don't want these; I want to get better."

Clint painfully climbed into the wheelchair, and we headed toward the exit. I could see his angry white knuckles as he held his crutches up while I wheeled him out. As we rounded the last corner past the emergency room doors, the young girl who had completed the intake process came around from behind us. She handed Clint a small piece of paper. "Don't look at this until you are outside," she whispered. "I'll get fired. Please don't get me in trouble." She stepped away and waved, raising her voice.

"Bye, Clint. I hope you feel better soon." With that, she disappeared around the corner.

I looked at Clint, and he tucked the piece of paper under his shirt. "That was weird," he muttered.

Leaving him at the exit doors, I went to get the car. Rain was coming down hard, and I was soaked by the time I got to the parking garage. In a few moments, my son was carefully climbing into the car beside me. What the hell had just happened? What was going on? It was like we were trapped in an episode of *The Twilight Zone*.

Between an Asian doctor whispering information into Clint's ear and someone else handing him a note on a small piece of paper, I was starting to wonder how deep this mystery went.

"What does the paper say?" I asked as soon as he was securely in the car.

"I was afraid to open it," he said, pulling it out from under his shirt. "It has a name and a phone number on it. That's all. Is it just another doctor?" He sounded utterly discouraged. "Who cares? I just want to die! I'm over this, and I have another surgery in a few weeks. Where is all of this going? I just want to die."

Glancing over at him, I thought about his pain being far more than physical. He was experiencing extraordinary emotional pain and mental anguish too. Cancer victims get an insurance code. Poisoned people do not.

"I'm going to figure this out. I promise," I told him, as I had been telling him since 2004—and I still meant it.

The rain seemed like it couldn't possibly pour down any harder, but it did, just as I kept thinking Clint couldn't take anymore—but he did. From what source did he draw his strength?

"Okay, Clint, we are home. Let me get the car in the garage. I don't want you to slip on those crutches and break your leg." He mumbled agreement as the garage door went up. "I love you. We will win. I promise we will win," I whispered.

I pulled the car into the garage, and Clint and I entered the house, hungry, exhausted, and essentially no better off than we had been at eight o'clock that morning. I had another bill to pay, and Clint had more pain.

It can't get any worse, I thought. Stupid, stupid thinking!

We walked into the basement, where Clint had been forced to stay, twenty-four/seven, since he couldn't climb stairs in his current state, to find it full of water. Clint's bedroom had two inches of water on the floor, and his carpet was soaked. His couch, dresser, and bed were swimming in water.

Clint couldn't help, and everything was wet. The water pressure was so intense coming down the hill against the house that it had eroded the concrete joints between the old basement and the addition that was put on the house twenty-some years earlier. Water was rolling in like a river. Clint's room didn't have a floor drain, so I had to move fast to save his stuff. It was a physical battle. We had not eaten all day. My reserves were long gone. I pulled myself together and went to work.

A neighbor came down and helped me do what could be done. We moved Clint upstairs for the time being. This was okay, except the upstairs shower wasn't a walk-in, neighborhood noise hurt his head, and sunshine through the window shades hurt his eyes.

Early Monday morning, I was on the phone, trying to find the doctor to whom we had been clandestinely referred. His name was Dr. Carl Fritzmeyer. He, along with Kara's real-life counterpart, agreed to allow me to use his real name here, but my attorney did not agree to any such thing.

They're good people. Dr. Fritzmeyer is a nutritionist with a practice called Body in Balance in Charleston. He answered his phone the first time I called. He answered as if he was expecting a challenge or as if he was ready for me. He sounded very sincere on the phone and completely surprised when I told him where I had gotten his name.

"I'm really busy," he said. "Let me see what I can do." He'd heard enough of my story to know Clint was in big trouble. "How about Wednesday morning around eight o'clock?" he asked.

Ecstatic, I thanked him and said goodbye. Did you notice the difference between him and the other doctors' offices? Did you notice the absence of a six-week wait? No waiting; we'd be seeing him in two days. Did you notice that I talked to the doctor himself? He didn't need a protective wall of overworked, hateful office women to screen his phone calls. The young woman at the hospital had given me his cell phone number. Dr. Fritzmeyer had had no idea who was calling him, yet he had answered the call.

Clint was still upstairs. It had been difficult, but we were making it work the best we could.

"Morning," he called as I tried to tiptoe to the shower. He was awake. He was always awake.

It was Wednesday, the day we were to go see Dr. Fritzmeyer, so there was no time for Clint to get into the chamber that day. Clint dragged himself out of his new bedroom with quite a bit of effort, looking like he'd been living on the street his entire life.

I was worried. Would this be another dead end with no answer, no medical reason for Clint's condition? Clint couldn't climb stairs. The only way to come and go from our house without stairs was via the back door from the den. Clint went around the house and down the hill, through the slippery grass, to the street. I picked him up there. Everything had become a struggle.

It would be another late night for me since I would be taking him to Beckley going home and then driving back to town, which was halfway back to Beckley again. *This had better be worth it,* I thought. Dr. Fritzmeyer didn't take insurance, so this would be out of pocket again. I was really worried about all the bills.

Clint moaned and groaned in pain as we traveled potholed Kanawha

Turnpike to Beckley. The road was a mess, in the process of being repaired in some spots and in need of attention in others. Clint keenly felt every bump.

"I'm so sorry," I said, cringing as I helped him out of the car. "I know that hurt. Let's hope this is worth the pain." I grabbed the medical reports from the past seven years while Clint grabbed his crutches.

He had been on crutches for almost a year. I worried about his knees, ankles, and shoulders. His body had been through a frightening amount of abuse. I worried about his hips lasting through whatever he was fighting. After all, we'd been doing things backward, addressing the symptoms but not finding and addressing the cause.

What was going to stop necrosis from happening again? No one seemed to be listening. I hoped Dr. Fritzmeyer would listen.

Dr. Fritzmeyer greeted us promptly. I liked his strong face and wide smile. He really wanted to know everything. First, he examined Clint. Then, he asked for the hormone tests from the prior year.

"How are you able to read the tests if the doctor that ordered them couldn't?" I asked. Dr. Fritzmeyer looked at me with respect; I could tell he understood the pain and frustration of my past seven years. I handed him a jam-packed three-inch binder containing Clint's medical records. He opened the test pages and scanned though the lines of information.

He touched Clint's arm and said, "I will do the best I can. There's a lot to fix. There's very little time."

He understood the entirety of the test results. He explained why Clint had no hormones and explained what it meant to Clint's body. Without hormones, the body shuts down.

This surprised me. I didn't know that hormones did so much. I heard him loud and clear. Clint's liver was pretty much gone. Without a functioning liver, there were no hormones. And without hormones, there's no resting body state. Without cholesterol, food digestion is nonexistent, which will cause a person to die a slow and painful death.

Dr. Fritzmeyer said the first thing we had to do was change Clint's diet. Proper food intake was the only way to fix our problem. A proper diet would help the liver and intestines.

He mentioned leaky gut syndrome and said that the supplements Clint was taking would never work without changing his diet to repair the gut.

"Diet and supplements work in tandem," the doctor explained. "For starters, Clint needs some blood tests."

Furthermore, Dr. Fritzmeyer knew where to send the urine collection kit that we had received from the emergency room. He told us he planned to call his friends around the country to ask for ideas. In the meantime, he gave Clint a diet plan, which was basically as follows:

Red beets
Greens (e.g., kale, collards, spinach, broccoli)
Protein (e.g., meat, fish, beans, nuts)
No sugar
No milk

We learned that calcium in milk carries the lead into the bones. The lead pushes out the calcium. Remember, the oversupply of calcium in Clint's blood tests that I previously mentioned? If Dr. Bio-Identity had done her homework, she might have understood why Clint's blood showed too much calcium. It's because the lead had moved in, and calcium was pushed out of the bones. Once the metals take over the body, lead makes the brain think it is calcium. The brain does a calcium exchange for the cheap imitation calcium, lead. Because of this, the bones begin the cellular death progression.

Sometime in the past few days, I had made contact with a chemist and asked him how to get out arsenic. He had said, "Eat raw garlic—lots and lots of raw clove garlic." When I asked about this, Dr. Fritzmeyer agreed. We had a plan.

"I am a nutritionist," Dr. Fritzmeyer explained right before we left. "I am a Western-licensed chiropractic doctor. I fix people by proper diets and lifestyle changes. It's not easy. It's not fast. That's the problem; you are nearly out of time." He looked at Clint. "I've never seen such a live dead person. I'm surprised you're still breathing! Every living organ in your body is malfunctioning. I have a feeling the metals are in your brain. I have never ever seen anything like you before. Frankly, you should be dead."

It seemed that medical professionals uttered that statement everywhere we went.

He then said, "Removing heavy metals from the body is a slow and extremely painful process. It's thought that as many years as the metals have ruled your functionality, that's how many years it will take to detoxify them out. It's a laborious process. The latest pain that you've experienced will be the first to let up. That pain will be worse than it was. You will have to experience each previous pain phase in reverse. Detoxification is not for the weak. There is no simple way to get this done. Since you have been sick for nearly ten years, I'm afraid it will take ten years to remove these metals. I'm just not so sure your body can live through it. If you are willing to go the distance, I'm in the game with you. There will be no pharmaceutical drugs to help, as they will cause more harm to your liver. No pain medications will help with the pain. What you have just gone through will be relived."

Clint was very silent as Dr. Fritzmeyer spoke. He just kept looking at me like he wasn't there anymore. He was just a shell covered in yellow skin and sunken, hollow eyes. He whispered, "What else can I do? I just won't die. So let's get this ship turning around."

We shook the doctor's hand and thanked him so many times that it was embarrassing. He told us that he would be in touch next week. We left more scared than we were upon arriving.

Clint continued to climb into the chamber twice a day. I kept trying to save my son's life. The reality set in that Clint might never go back to work. We both realized that it would have to wait. His right hip still needed to be decompressed. Clint was working every single minute, strengthening his left hip in preparation for July 11.

During the next visit, Dr. Fritzmeyer suggested that we call the Social Security Disability office. "Clint is sicker than you know," he explained. "He will not be going back to work for a long time, if ever. You're going to need help. Have you contacted the Bureau of Worker's Compensation?"

So much to do, so little time, I thought.

I went online to begin the disability paperwork. I searched for a disability attorney or a work injury attorney.

Several personal injury attorneys looked at the case. I wrote to the Freedom of Information Office in Chicago and requested a violation report concerning ULTRA. The problem is, you have to ask for certain years. You have to know what you don't know in hopes of getting what you need to know. I sent the request and received a large box in return for my money spent. There were pages and pages of violations—just for the few years I requested. This proved to be a waste of my time, as no one I contacted cared or could see a connection between those reports and Clint's symptoms.

Before and after we had made that trip to CAMC's emergency room, I had been calling every toxicologist doctor in Charleston. I called Saint Albans Group Health in Saint Albans and talked to Marliss at some point that spring.

She had said that Dr. Boshaft did not treat chronic patients. I called Marliss again, on or around June 9. That time, she said she would have Dr. Boshaft call us. Ten days later, Dr. Boshaft called.

I kept Excel spreadsheets to track conversations that Clint or I had with different contacts. Here is one—from Clint's perspective—that will set the tone for the rest of this story:

June 20, 2011

9:47 a.m.—Our house phone rang. "Hello, this Dr. Barnes from the Saint Albans Group. I got your information from Marliss Burke. I want to talk with you about your health issues. Can you come in here for an appointment?"

"I'm on another line right now, requesting my medical records," Clint told him.

"I have about twenty minutes to talk right now. I'm in between patients," Dr. Barnes said.

Clint was confused as to why this Dr. Barnes would be calling our house at 9:47 a.m., so he told him he would have to call him back.

Clint called his newly hired worker's compensation attorney, along with his new personal injury attorney, to ask them if it was okay to talk with this unknown doctor.

11:00 a.m.—BWC (Bureau of Worker's Compensation) attorney George Cosby wanted Dr. Barnes's number so he could call him.

12:30 p.m.—Personal injury attorney Mark Otiose gave Clint the go-ahead to talk to this doctor.

1:11 p.m.—Our house phone rang. "Hello, this is Dr. Damen Boshaft from the Saint Albans Group. I got your name from Marliss Burke and Dr. Barnes."

Clint asked, "Who are you?"

Dr. Boshaft said, "I am the director of Saint Albans Group." Clint noted the phone number on the caller ID. Dr. Boshaft was on Otiose's list of toxicologists that Clint needed to see. This all seemed okay. Dr. Boshaft started off asking questions about the job, where Clint had been, and what he had worked on in the ULTRA plant.

Clint stopped him to ask, "Why does this matter if you are the doctor?"

Dr. Boshaft said, "I know that plant inside and out, and I know what they do."

This made sense to Clint. He figured this would help the doctor know with what he had come in contact and help point him in the right direction for a solution to his health situation. But the conversation didn't go that way. Dr. Boshaft was more interested in names of the ULTRA supervisors, what Clint worked on, and who told him what to do. Clint kept telling Dr. Boshaft that he was in the maintenance department and that he did all kinds of jobs all over the entire plant.

Clint told me that he asked Dr. Boshaft three or four times, "Are you a real doctor, or do you work for ULTRA? What's the deal?"

Dr. Boshaft just repeated, "I am the director of Saint Albans Group."

Dr. Boshaft then began asking Clint medical health questions, and Clint listed all the multiple problems he'd had since 2004.

In fewer than ten minutes, Dr. Boshaft announced, "It's not arsine gas or arsenic poisoning. I will send you release-of-medical-record forms. I need to know everything since birth: illnesses, broken bones, childhood issues ..." The list went on and on. The conversation lasted an hour and a half.

I had called Saint Albans Group Toxicology numerous times in the past. Every single time I had been told there was no such thing as chronic poisoning. They refused to give Clint an appointment. I called them last Thursday when WV Poison Center had told Clint to go to the emergency room in order to gain access to CAMC's toxicology department. On that Thursday, Saint Albans said no, Clint could not see a doctor. (Much later, I found out that Dr. Boshaft was the doctor who ran CAMC's toxicology department until he moved to Saint Albans. I also found out, months later that Dr. Boshaft was working with ULTRA, writing protocols for arsenic poisoning emergencies while Clint worked there.)

Why would a doctor spend ninety minutes talking to someone who was not his patient? Let's face it; I couldn't get Clint's doctors to spend five minutes on the phone with me. Clint's doctors had Clint's insurance card. What doctor works for free? Did Dr. Boshaft? I highly doubt it. Something was wrong with this picture.

Clint asked Dr. Boshaft, "Why do you need to know what happened before 2004? I was healthy. Nothing was wrong. Why do you need to know about a broken hand in junior high? Do you work for ULTRA? Are you interested in my health or the health of ULTRA?"

Dr. Boshaft lied at this point and said, "I am not associated with ULTRA. You would have had to have blood in your urine to have been poisoned with arsine. You would have been deathly sick that same day if you came in contact with it."

Clint told him, "I repaired that machine, and it must have had some chemical in it that I came in contact with. I need to know what that chemical was. I have a twenty-four-hour urine test that CAMC Emergency sent home. I have no idea what to do with it. It is supposedly to see if I have arsenic in my urine. However, I have called several labs, and no one has ever heard of it. Have you?"

Dr. Boshaft told Clint he had never heard of a twenty-four-hour urine test.

Dr. Boshaft was a highly respected toxicologist. He had published papers, yet he didn't know about this test?

Clint told Dr. Boshaft about his next surgery. He asked him about testing his bone chips. Dr. Boshaft told Clint that the bone chips would not test positive for arsenic. The conversation ended with Dr. Boshaft's determination that Clint was not poisoned. His symptoms were not caused by ULTRA.

They said goodbye. Dr. Boshaft had completely checked out Clint over the phone and decided he was not poisoned. That was about a two-hour consultation for no pay. Who does that?

Clint and I decided that Dr. Boshaft's was not a safe place to go. Something felt wrong with that phone conversation. Either way, the intake paperwork that Dr. Boshaft was going to send never arrived. Dr. Boshaft had been fishing. *Fishing for what?* I wondered.

Without telling me, Clint spent his days harassing ULTRA in Dallas. He was digging for information, just like I had asked him to do. We needed to figure out what we didn't know.

It was the end of June, and I had finally finished filling out the Social Security paperwork online.

Clint was home alone when the phone rang.

"I'm from the Social Security office in Charleston," a man said. "I need more information to complete your disability request. May I ask you a few questions?"

"Go ahead," Clint said. He was confused. This was the second person to call him asking for more information.

The man asked Clint what happened and the dates of the events—all the usual questions. All of a sudden, in the middle of the conversation, the caller's voice got very low. "I will call you back from a different line. Make sure you answer the phone. Answer on the first ring. I need to call you on my cell phone."

Clint answered on the first ring. "What's going on?" he asked.

"I'm sorry. I only have a minute. Listen to me—I have to get back upstairs before someone notices I'm gone. I talk to so many of you, many construction guys that are sick just like you ... Find Dr. Marcel Tiens. Find him now. He has an office in Falling Rock and has been spending a lot of time in Ohio, trying to save the people who were poisoned by Fernald. He's your only hope. He can get out the metal. I have to go back inside. I'll call you back. Find Dr. Tiens!"

Clint hung up, and moments later, the home phone rang again. The Social Security representative continued the call with Clint as if he had never called him from his cell phone. When the conversation ended, Clint immediately called me. He talked like he could explode at any minute, telling me about the phone call. He could hardly catch his breath. I wrote down everything he said.

I looked up Dr. Tiens's phone number and called asking him—no, *begging* him—to see Clint. He told me to drop off my son's medical records on Thursday night, July 7.

July 2011

In the midst of this drama, more was added to the mix.

I called every agency I could think of to find out what had happened at the ULTRA plant in Pennsylvania. Finally, someone in the hazmat division told me about the things that happened. Bad things. He told me to search online for a newspaper article published in the *Pittsburgh Post-Gazette*.

On July, 4, 2011, while I everyone else was celebrating the holiday, I was on the internet, searching for something else I needed to know. This is what I found:

Chemical accident injures man

By Steve Perkins

Staff Writer

Tuesday, August 12, 2008

KDKA-TV reports that following a potentially deadly accident overnight, Air Care transported a Cranberry Township worker to a St. Clair Hospital. A Hazmat team was summoned to the ULTRA plant, where the worker may have been exposed to the potentially deadly chemical, arsenic.

According to Cranberry Township Fire Chief Peter Gates, officials from across the area responded at 1 a.m. to assist a worker who had been trapped in a storage container that formerly held chemicals, including arsenic. The man was flown to St. Clair Hospital in Pittsburgh around three o'clock this morning.

Gates said that the measures taken were purely precautionary. "When we arrived, the victim was out of the tank and site workers were rendering first aid. The tank was empty and it was undergoing maintenance," Gates said. "More is being made of this than it deserves. The tank once contained arsenic was cleaned out some time ago." Gates reported that the victim, who still remains unidentified, was still at St. Clair Hospital undergoing tests. "He's alert and should be all right," said Gates.

This is the second incident at ULTRA, which makes circuit boards for computers, since January 2008. A chemical spill at the plant on January 5 sent twenty employees to the hospital.

ULTRA officials could not be reached for comment regarding the incident.

The piece concluded with contact information—a phone number and email address—for the reporter.

I called the *Pittsburgh Post-Gazette* and connected with Steve Perkins's desk. A man who identified himself as Richard Wilson answered the phone.

"May I please talk to Steve Perkins?" I asked.

"He's gone," he said.

"Where did he go? I need to talk to him about an article that was published in this newspaper in 2008. It's about a chemical accident at the ULTRA plant in Pittsburgh, Pennsylvania."

"Well, he no longer works here, so you can't," he snapped.

"How long did he last after this article was printed?" I asked, now in an equally nasty voice. "Let me guess—about six months?"

"That's about right," he admitted. "But the article you're referring to isn't the reason he was let go. He had issues."

"I'll bet he did. Do you want to cover a real story? Do you want to get discovered? Maybe that's what Steve wanted when he stumbled into this mess. Go down to ULTRA. See what's going on. See what went on. Research the fact that the governor paid them to come here for his political needs after ULTRA was thrown out of Washington State. You'll find out that they left Pennsylvania without fulfilling their promises and never repaid the tax abatement money. Write to the Freedom of Information office in Chicago and see the hundreds of EPA violations they had in Pennsylvania. They're still at the plant cleaning up! What are they cleaning up? Don't you want to know? Maybe the internet articles I found are wrong. Maybe I'm wrong. But something is wrong. There's something here. Don't you want to know?"

"Lady, you have no idea what you are getting into. Steve was crazy, and so are you," he said dismissively.

A few months later, when I looked for that article again, it was completely gone from the internet. I have copies, lots of copies, of that article and a few others that can't be found anywhere online anymore.

The timeline regarding Dr. Boshaft, the Social Security representative, and the newspaper article were all only a couple of weeks apart.

On Thursday night, July 7, I drove to Falling Rock to drop off Clint's three-inch jam-packed three-ring binder of medical records to Dr. Tiens.

Clint had surgery scheduled four days later. Exhausted, I struggled to get through another day. I wondered how much more Clint's body could take, and I was running out of time and ideas.

With Falling Rock in my rearview mirror, I answered a call on my cell phone.

"Mom!" Clint shouted in a panic. "Dr. Boshaft just called and yelled at me. He said that I'm going to die and nobody will help me! He says no toxicologist in the country will see me. He told me he will make sure of that. He said—" My phone went dead. Service wasn't great where I was and didn't come back for several excruciating minutes. Finally, the phone rang again. Sounding even more panicked, Clint repeated what he had already told me until I lost service again.

Entries from my records are as follows:

On 7/5/2011

Clint called Dr. Boshaft and asked what happened to the paperwork that he promised to mail on June 20, 2011. He left a message on his answering machine earlier that day. Clint told him NIOSH told him to call and ask Dr. Boshaft if he is a toxicologist because they have never heard of anyone diagnosing a person—especially when the person is not a patient—over the phone.

They also said because he talked to Clint for two hours, he should be willing to see him and send the information he promised.

Dr. Boshaft didn't call back.

On 7/6/2011

Clint called CAMC. They told him that the people that specialize in toxic poisoning are in Saint Albans Group. Clint left another message on Dr. Boshaft's answering machine.

Remember, I had just found the article about the chemical spill at ULTRA and had really begun shaking some trees on July 5. Clint was doing his tree shaking as well. Here is what happened.

On 7/7/2011

Dr. Boshaft called our home on July 7, 2011, at 5:50 p.m. from his cell phone. He claimed he had mailed the new patient paperwork on June 21. Clint told him that we had not gotten anything from him.

Dr. Boshaft started to give Clint his email address but changed his mind before finishing it.

Here is how the conversation went:

Dr. B. said, "You and your mom need to stop calling and bothering me because you don't have arsine poisoning."

Clint told him about the newspaper article that we found on the internet, dated August 12, 2008.

Dr. B. replied, "That article was a lie, and that reporter was fired. Stop looking things up about ULTRA! Things on the internet and in newspaper articles are not true." Another doctor that didn't want us to use the internet.

Clint said, "My mom called the *Post-Gazette* to talk to Steve Perkins. Richard answered the desk line and told my mom Steve was fired. She asked Richard how many toes Steve stepped on when he released this story."

Dr. B. answered, "Perkins was fired because that accident didn't happen. He lied! You will not find any records of that ever happening because it never happened."

Clint answered, "That is just not true. I have the article right here."

"You and your mom need to stop reading stuff on the internet because I am the expert on arsine," Dr. B. said. Abruptly, the phone connection was lost.

At 6:02 p.m., Dr. Boshaft called back, cursing angrily. "You and your mom need to stop harassing me and ULTRA! Stop looking up arsine or anything else on ULTRA."

Clint replied, "It sounds to me like you work for ULTRA, not—"

The cell phone went dead again.

At 6:10 p.m., Dr. Boshaft called back. He was more than angry this time.

Dr. B: "You don't know who you are fucking with. Stop digging up information on ULTRA! You and your mom do not have enough resources to pursue ULTRA or me. You do not know who you are messing with. By the time you find out what is poisoning you, it will be too late, and you will have cancer or be dead from the poison. We [*meaning ULTRA and him?*] will drag this out. Once you have cancer, you will never have a case. Don't fucking ever call me again. No one in Charleston will ever help you."

Clint: "Why are you getting so upset about me saying things about ULTRA? Do you work for them? Are they paying you?"

Dr. Boshaft hung up.

Obviously, that was a train wreck of a night for Clint and me. A few weeks later, the following letter arrived at my house.

[masthead]
18 July 2011

Clint Marshall
[INSIDE ADDRESS]

Dear Mr. Marshall:

I'm sorry our conversation went so poorly.

I'm not certain what happened to the documents I sent via email.

I've enclosed copies of the stuff I found along with several forms to authorize release of information. When you've completed the forms, contact the office. I will tell my staff to watch for your FAX and ensure that I receive it.

Sincerely,
[signature]
Damien Boshaft [signature] [contact information]

Clint was still staying upstairs because of the damage to the basement. I was trying desperately to move him downstairs before the July 11 decompression procedure. Clint couldn't do the work. He knew what needed to be done but didn't have the ability to physically do it.

So Clint leaned on his crutches and watched my friends do his job. He instructed them on what needed to be done. He told them how far to drill out the crumbled concrete wall and how to pack a waterproof mixture of concrete back into the drilled-out foundation. His job-hopping, learn-by-doing-construction college education was being utilized.

Clint was the foreman on this job. I was the cleanup crew.

At the end of my day, sometime between dinner, some client work, and my shower, I would clean up concrete dust. Scott, one of my many clients, would come over to hammer drill out the walls. Garin helped put in insulation after the walls were repaired. Scott and a buddy hung the drywall. The clock was ticking. With only three days to spare, I quickly painted the walls, and we finished Clint's room.

Finally, I found an internet site about testing for heavy metals in the human body. Everywhere I had called since 2004 said that Clint would not be alive if he had toxic welding products or residual arsenic still in him from seven years ago. They all told me that the body naturally cleanses these toxins from itself. If Clint had really done what I explained to them without using a respirator or clean air supply, he would have immediately died from that high concentration of exposure.

Yet he did, and he was still alive—if you could call his current life "living." Denial from government agencies seems to be the general rule of thumb as I strove to find the answers that we needed.

At four thirty in the morning on July 11, 2011, we headed out the door to his second decompression procedure. Dr. Khanna had said he had to do the next decompression as soon as possible.

This day was a repeat of the left hip decompression. I weighed less and had more stress.

Clint was very sick. His bladder never ever stopped twitching. He still had a twenty-four/seven symptom that mimicked a urinary tract infection. Nothing had changed much in regard to the over body burden.

As usual, we met with Dr. Khanna before the surgery. He was distant and seemed angry when we talked. He stayed coldly professional and chose his words carefully. When the procedure was finished, the relationship with Lighthouse Orthopedics was finished as well.

I really don't remember much of that day. As the metals in Clint mixed, causing his body to be a giant chemistry experiment, my exhausted brain was having serious problems connecting the dots of my days' activities.

The entire time Clint was in the operating room, I replayed that month's drama in my mind, trying to separate truth from emotion in order to come up with a game plan. *Think, think, think! What is going on here?* What did I need to know that I didn't know in order to figure this out? *Come on, brain—kick into overdrive. Do your thing!*

I had contacted the Centers for Disease Control in Atlanta, Georgia, sometime in the past two years. I had asked them if they could test Clint for metal poisoning. They told me that I had to know which metal I was looking for before they could order the test. I would have to pay per metal, and it would become very expensive. They ended the conversation with *sorry.* At that point, I had no idea what I was looking for. I just knew that I was looking. Looking and hoping for the next door to open. I had no idea where I was going.

The medical world does not give Reliable Data, Inc. unqualified respect, at least not on the internet. This company claimed to be able to test hair samples and identify the heavy metals in the human body. I was beginning my journey into the crazy side of figuring out this puzzle. But Reliable Data was the only site that offered me any hope for answers—and we were already on our way down that slippery slope of not being understood.

But after all, Georgia had told me that I needed to find out what we were looking for before they could help me!

When we got home from the decompression procedure, I ordered Reliable Data's kit. It arrived five days later. Following the kit's instructions, I prepared the sample and mailed it the next morning.

Clint had come home from the hospital prepared to die. His body was shutting down. By this time, most of the metals in Clint had found safe haven in his bones, brain, and soft tissue. Hair was no longer a true test of his actual levels. The lead had already pushed the calcium out of his bones and moved right in. I was later told that was why he had such an extreme amount of calcium in his blood. He no longer had any in his bones. Other metals had moved into his soft tissue. That is what caused his pelvic-floor disease. The metals caused knots in the muscles in his pelvic floor, and eventually they lost their strength, creating the spasms of pain. Other metals were in his spine, climbing up into his head. They caused swelling that was responsible for his unexplained back problems. When the metals made it into the brain, the headaches and vision issues began. Neurons in his brain could no longer communicate with his cells, and cellular death followed. This inability to communicate was called white noise. The red blood cells could not carry enough oxygen. This caused necrosis. The white blood cells were not told when to purge. These white blood cells built up in the joints, causing arthritis and painful swelling. This caused

Clint's hips to lock up and hurt. He had the arthritic hips of a fifty-eight-year-old. The white blood cells collecting in his elbows caused them to become immobile for five to ten minutes at a stretch. Clint's lymph nodes were so overly congested with dead white blood cells that the circulation was cut off around his groin area, causing testicular pain. His boggy prostate was because the white blood cells and microscopic metal ions were trapped in the prostate tissue. His collapsed urethra was caused by the intense swelling of his urinary tract.

I did not learn all this until 2011. It was an extremely painful education. Yet Clint and I have not been allowed to discuss this with his Western-licensed doctors. I searched Clint's current situations and symptoms as they appeared. I found theories on holistic cures on the internet. I know which ones worked and absolutely know the pharmaceutical drugs did nothing positive. Once the metals began to be detoxified, Clint's unexplainable symptoms began to disappear. Gone!

After the phone call with Dr. Boshaft, I decided that I needed to get away from Charleston. I needed to find a toxicologist out of town. On July 20 at 11:45 a.m., I called an occupational therapy clinic in Chicago and spoke directly to Dr. Barston. After listening to my story, he said he would see Clint.

"How soon can you send the records? Does he have insurance?" he asked. I gave him the information. I told him about arsenic exposure and the tank work that I believe caused it.

Then I made the mistake of mentioning ULTRA.

About two hours after my conversation with Dr. Barston at 1:55 p.m. the same day, Clint got a phone call on our home phone. Clint recounted it to me later that night after I got home.

"Something strange happened today, Mom. The phone rang, and someone was there but would not talk. I wrote down the number. It's a Dallas area code. I tried to call it back, but it's one of those outgoing-only lines."

My stomach did a complete flip. At 2:52 p.m., I had received a phone call from Dr. Barston, saying that he had changed his mind and could not see Clint. He told me he thought it would be better for everyone if we stayed local.

Was that phone call to see if Clint was still alive and looking for help? I thought. *I can't get into that right now. More enemies are creating a new front for me to battle while Clint is still knocking on death's door.*

We need a toxicologist to help Clint. I'm smart enough to know that I'm not smart enough to cure Clint on my own. We're not doctors. West Virginia Poison Center told me that I need a toxicologist to get this out of my son.

Resuming the search for a toxicologist, I contacted West Virginia Health in Lewisburg, where a neurologist toxicologist practiced.

"Clint, we're in luck," I said. "I've made an appointment for you to see a toxicologist in Lewisburg. This will be so much better than going all the way to Chicago. Things are looking up! Your surgeries were all successful. Things are going your way." As Clint was getting sicker every day, I was determined to stress to him, as well as to myself, the positive things that were happening. I couldn't fall apart; I didn't have time. Determination was the only thing I had left. My heart and brain were crushed with fear of losing this battle. But I feigned optimism for Clint's sake.

The appointment, set for September 7, was a very long two months away. Telling myself that the best doctors often have long wait times, I gathered all of Clint's records to send on a memory stick and spent hours scanning and saving the records to the external drive. In two days, everything was in the mail.

"I have a good feeling about this," I told Clint.

"I hope, Mom," he responded weakly. "I hope."

I was on the internet, constantly searching sites that reported EPA violations. I found many items regarding ULTRA's lack of environmental respect.

Much had happened over the past few months.

While we waited for the appointment with the toxicologist, we had a postsurgery appointment with Dr. Khanna.

"I bought a hyperbaric chamber, and Clint gets into it two times a day," I mentioned to Dr. Khanna. "What's your opinion regarding oxygen therapy?"

"I have no idea," Dr. Khanna replied offhandedly.

"Do you think Clint has necrosis from being a pipe fitter?" I asked.

"Now that you mention it," he said, with a thoughtful roll of his eyes upward and to the right, "most of my AVN patients are welders and pipe fitters between the ages of twenty-four and forty."

He's just now putting that together—really? "What do you think that means?" I asked.

"I don't know. I really haven't thought about it. That's not my area," he said briskly, obviously wanting to end the conversation.

"There has to be a connection, right?" I pressed persistently. *What's it going to hurt?*

He gave me an irritated look. "I don't know. It's not my area! You need to find a toxicologist."

"Know any?" I asked, trying not to smirk.

"Can't say I do. See you in a few weeks. Keep up the good work, Clint." With that, he was gone.

Dr. Fritzmeyer, with Body in Balance, was diligently—perhaps desperately—searching for supplements and diet ideas to save Clint's liver and intestines and, in turn, his adrenal glands. I too kept working and researching.

Attorney Otiose was working on Clint's case. He had represented the two men who were injured in what I figured was the previously mentioned accident of 2008. He never confirmed that for me, but that remains my assumption. I had a connection with someone who was related to an employee of Otiose. She told me that he won that case. It would have been impossible to lose. It was acute poisoning. There was no denying where those men were injured. Clint's case was different. His body had been dying over the course of seven years.

"You don't have a case," Otiose told me a few months later. He explained that a discovery rule is part of the statute of limitations for personal injury cases. Companies are protected from lawsuits when the injury is reported more than two years after the onset of the first symptom. By the time the employee figures out why he or she is sick and believes it's because of a company, it may well be past the two-year mark of discovery, and the worker cannot file a claim. When Clint first became sick, I knew he was suffering from poisoning. I felt for sure it was from his job, but I could not find any time to think about a lawsuit. This law, once again, was all about protecting the offender, not safeguarding the disposable worker. I didn't have time to prove my thoughts.

Dr. Boshaft was on Otiose's referral list. Otiose represented the other two men and had a direct connection with Dr. Boshaft. Dr. Boshaft had told Clint that ULTRA's pockets were way deeper than mine and that Clint would never find any help in Charleston. He had said Clint and I had no power against ULTRA and that Clint would be dead before a lawsuit ever went to court. It seemed like there was something in this that I needed to understand. But I had to stick to the important task: saving Clint. I smelled a rat.

I contacted another firm in Michigan, and they agreed to look at the case. After a couple of months reviewing my box of evidence, their story was this: "The wife of one of that firm's partners died from cancer, and he took a well-deserved leave of absence". Clint's case was thrown out. With a partner out on leave, they didn't have time to go up against ULTRA. Were they afraid of ULTRA?

That ended my search for the personal injury case. I didn't have the time or energy for it.

Dr. Boshaft, one; Peggy, zero, I thought.

At that point, we were working with our second worker's

compensation attorney. At that time, ULTRA was a Pennsylvania company. Century Construction was in West Virginia and had its assets in a different corporation. There was nothing to get. I was working between two states and two companies that were determined not to give us what we needed. Clint was sick and dying, and no one could be held responsible to help or give us the information we needed for him to get well.

Ten days after Clint's last hip surgery, he climbed into the car. "That surgery was brutal," he said. "Hip decompression is far worse than osteoarthritis surgery."

We were on our way to see the newest worker's compensation and Social Security disability attorney, whose office was on fifth floor of a building in downtown Charleston. Every single bump drove Clint into another pain spasm.

"I'm sorry. I'm sorry," I murmured repeatedly, cringing in sympathy as Clint moaned and cried out in pain. "Here—I'll drop you off at the door. Let me park the car, and I'll be right in. Try to find some place to sit down."

When I finally met Clint upstairs, he looked like he had just returned home from a war zone. The attorney ushered us into a room with a long dark wooden table, and we all sat down. The sun was coming in the window, and I zoned out.

This was my new problem. If I sat down any place other than in front of my computer, I fell asleep from sheer exhaustion.

Clint told his story to the attorney, and I wanted to let him tell it. Clint needed to tell it without my help. He had lived it. *And I relive it every time he repeats it.* I tried not to listen, as it had become extremely difficult for me.

The attorney kept looking my way. *Probably astonished that a mother could fall asleep while her dying son tells his story,* I thought. Through my half-closed eyes, I could see him looking at me, and I didn't care. That was how I'd chosen to cope with the day. I was exhausted to the point of physical pain from constantly seeking a way to save my son.

I drifted off and was heading down a wasp-infested road, where the stings kept getting more numerous and painful, and the allergic reaction became increasingly deadly.

As Clint became sicker, he became aggressively confused. He tended to repeat the same thing over and over again.

I was suffering from fight-or-flight. Some days I was good at being patient, as I was scared and filled with doubt. Sometimes Clint was loud and difficult when I said something he didn't want to hear or believe. This would activate my fight response, and we would battle. On such a day, I might scream at him, "Go away!"

I felt really bad about it when I snapped, but at such moments, I had nothing left to give. The thinker of great solutions had left the building.

As I heard his story in the background of my thoughts, I felt terrible for everything that I had missed from his first day on this earth. Maybe I could have done something better. Maybe I should have known more. *Isn't that what I am trying to do now?* I thought. *I am trying to know something that I do not know in order to prevent something that I fear will be a very bad end to this story. Stop!* I told myself. *Stop thinking!*

When Clint had finished telling his story, the attorney said, "I have never heard of such a thing! Your medical history is extensive. I'm afraid it's going to be impossible to prove any of this, let alone organize it into a case. No one goes to work for seven years in the condition you are in. No one could do that. You truly are *the last American cowboy.*"

Hearing those words, my head kicked back into life. *That is the truest statement I've heard in a really long time,* I thought.

That attorney tried for over a year to make a case for us. It never happened.

Dr. Boshaft, two; Peggy, zero, I thought.

Clint was working out as hard as he could to repair his hips. However, try as he might, his hips couldn't support his body to work out effectively.

Lighthouse had fallen apart. They had no idea how to rehabilitate Clint. Instead of being honest and treating us like members of a team, they pulled away further and stopped returning phone calls.

I decided to take over my son's therapy. Dr. Khanna had become useless. All my great thoughts and praise for Lighthouse died. The lighthouse went dark.

I called Roper Hospital's physical therapy department to ask if Clint could go there to use their warm water pool. They agreed but said they would need a prescription from Lighthouse. I called Dr. Khanna and asked him to send one over. He did as I asked but without any instructions. The therapist at Roper tried to help Clint, but in the absence of doctor's instructions, she couldn't help him much or for long. She would send notes regarding his progress. Dr. Khanna never responded to any of her requests for help.

I had dropped off Clint's medical records to Dr. Tiens on the first of July. "Come on Clint, let's go. It's our day with Dr. Tiens," I called down the stairs.

Clint, still on crutches, hobbled out the basement door. Thank God he was back in his room. He came out of the garage, got into the car, and off we went.

From the corner of my eye, I glimpsed him sitting there. *Dear Lord,* I prayed, *make something good happen tonight.* Having lost about forty-five pounds, Clint was down to 157 pounds. He still was not sleeping.

Dr. Fritzmeyer's diet plan seemed to be making a *small* difference. It had been very slow-going, though.

Clint's bladder continued to mimic having an infection, as it had for seven years.

"We're here," I said when we reached Dr. Tiens's office.

"Great," he said in a sad, worried voice.

Clint was starting to have more issues with his memory. He repeated himself more and more. As the metals took over the neuron communication center in his brain, it became more difficult for me to successfully communicate to him what we were doing and why it might improve his health. He became more pitiful and childlike with each passing day.

We walked into Dr. Tiens's office, which reminded me of doctors' offices I used to go to as a child: simple, nothing too sterile-looking. I noticed Doctor of the Year awards, for many years back, hanging on the walls. It looked like Marcel Tiens had never missed a year.

Clint met Dr. Tiens and his nurse (and wife). Nurse Roberta sat in with us as Clint began his seven-year story. The telling takes hours. Dr. Tiens never interrupted. He never looked at his watch or shuffled paperwork with a nervous look. He listened to the very end.

"Well, Clint," he began, "you have been through a lot in your short life. I'm not sure what I can do for you. There are so many issues; I just don't know."

That's when I started to cry. I hardly ever cry, and I *never* cry in public. I am a warrior, and warriors do *not* cry. They fight. But then and there, I cried.

Nurse Roberta looked at me with empathy. "You have to try," she murmured to her husband. "You have to do something."

Dr. Tiens sighed. After thinking a moment, he said, "Maybe we can try EDTA chelation therapy, a process by which metal ions in the body are bound to a chelating agent and excreted from the body. EDTA, or ethylenediaminetetraacetic acid, is a type of chelating agent. You would receive EDTA infusions. My concern is that you may not be strong enough to live through it. You have to know that, going in. It could either save you—or finish you off. Do you understand?" He paused, swallowed, and then said, "Your liver is 90 percent dead and may never regenerate. I've never seen anything like your condition. You should be dead, and you will be, if we don't do something."

Clint and I knew we had no other choice. We could either go with Dr.

Tiens's plan, or start planning Clint's funeral.

Connecting with Dr. Tiens proved to be excellent. There was a physical therapist in his building who'd had hip surgeries himself. Clint asked Dr. Khanna to send a prescription to that facility, but strangely, Dr. Khanna did not respond.

The physical therapist, Tim, decided to help rebuild Clint's hips without the prescription. Tim had had the same surgeries as Clint. He was an amateur cyclist who liked to climb mountains. This connection was exactly what I had been praying for. Clint really liked Tim too, which was a big help. My son's hips began to show improvement in strength and flexibility. Remember ... Clint and I were cash-only customers.

August 2011

On August 16, 2011, Clint and I went back to see Dr. Khanna for Clint's six-week postprocedural appointment. Clint was tired, sick, and exhausted. His hips checked out fine, according to Dr. Khanna. Otherwise, Dr. Khanna didn't have much to say. But I did.

"Dr. Khanna," I started firmly, "have you thought any more about the heavy-metal poison theory and AVN connection? I really wish you would've let me have those bone chips. It was such a waste to let them go when I really need to know what is in his bones."

Dr. Khanna was very guarded and seemed nervous about my reference to avascular necrosis. But he surprised me when he spoke. "I did have the bone chips tested," he said.

My ears perked up. *Maybe he can tell me what is in his bones!* I thought, but the thought was short-lived.

"I had the bones checked for steroid and alcohol abuse."

In complete disbelief, it was my turn to look at him like he had two heads. "*What*? You tested his bones for *your* needs but ignored your patient's needs?" I was furious.

Dr. Khanna looked straight at me, longer than normal. He just stared at me. My inner thoughts were so loud; it would not have much surprised me to learn I had screamed them aloud. *You arrogant son of a bitch!*

"So what did you find? Find any steroids? Find any alcohol?" I asked tightly through clenched teeth.

"No, I didn't. But I'm very concerned as to why this happened. I want Clint to have his blood tested to see if he is carrying any of the genes that are being recognized as transporters of heavy metals."

I sat there in sheer shock, my muscles twitching like a prize fighter before the Golden Glove fight. I really wanted to punch him.

"My wife is an oncologist/hematologist," he explained.

Why is he sharing this with me now? I wondered.

"I need to know if Clint is carrying any of those genes. It's extremely important for his future."

What future? He is dying, I thought in frustration and dismay. But then I had another glimmer of hope spring into my mind. I think Dr. Khanna had Clint's bone chips tested for heavy metals, as I'd asked. I think Dr. Khanna knew that Clint was dying from TILT. I think he was not allowed to tell us what he found.

I thanked Dr. Khanna for thinking outside his comfort zone.

Dr. Khanna asked Clint if he could give his cell phone number to his wife. Clint and I exchanged startled glances. This was highly unusual.

Why didn't he just give us her office number? We could call it and hear that we had to wait six weeks for an appointment. Then we would finally go to the appointment and be treated like we were crazy people, right?

Clint gave Dr. Khanna his cell phone number and agreed to the plan. The very next day, Dr. Khanna called. She instructed Clint to go to an off-site office in our neighborhood to have his blood drawn. Clint did not then—nor did he ever—meet her. Frankly, since our insurance paid for the tests, we never needed to know whose name was on the order.

A couple of weeks later, Dr. Khanna called from her cell phone with the test results. We were caught off guard when she called after office hours. We had hope that she was different from the countless Western medicine-practicing doctors we had seen in the past.

She told Clint that here was no medical reason for him to have necrosis. She needed more blood and wanted to know more. Although he suspected it was more for her research than in service to solving his precarious health mystery, Clint agreed and went back to the same office.

The office staff was very curious as to why Clint was having these tests done. The blood orders were different from most. When he told them his story, their questions stopped. Somehow, these results were back in less than two weeks. Again, Dr. Khanna called from her cell phone, after hours, to talk with Clint. Again, she said there was nothing wrong with his blood. Since she had no further explanations, she said goodbye. This concluded another confusing saga in a long line of unexplained happenstance.

The test results had come back negative for all the genes (identifiable at the time) that transport metals. Clint didn't have any. He didn't have a single cancer cell in him. What he did have was the gene that makes him a bleeder. Is that something Lighthouse should have been aware of before they ever cut him open? That would have been useful information. I wondered if Dr. Khanna got that important piece of information from his wife. I wondered if he thought about the fact that Lighthouse performed four invasive, heavy-bleeding operations on Clint, and after the fact, they found out he has the gene that makes him a bleeder. Lucky for all, that gene was still asleep.

In mid-July I had found an article on the internet about a major university study concerning heavy metal and a gene called Slc39a8. A paragraph from the article read, "Studying low doses of cadmium in mice, researchers found that the gene Slc39a8 transports cadmium to the testes, causing the tissue to die."

Clint constantly said his testicles felt like someone was standing on him wearing high heels. I wondered, *Is that what testes feel like as they die? I wondered if the hair test would show Clint had cadmium in him.*

I emailed the professor to see if I could get Clint into the study, but the researcher was not interested. He said he had his "own people."

He suggested that I have some blood tests done and send him the results. I figured the tests were expensive, and if he wasn't interested enough to help me get those done, he wouldn't accept Clint after he received the test results, so I let it drop. Besides, Clint had just had blood drawn a short time ago and tests supposedly showed nothing. But I had to wonder. These tests were not for Clint's benefit, so who could say if they told us the truth?

Why should I waste valuable time continuing to attempt to force open the gate to the Western medical community that was determined to see my son die?

Dr. Tiens wanted to begin the EDTA infusion therapy at the end of September. But first he wanted to save Clint's liver. He wanted to give Clint a little more time to stay on Dr. Fritzmeyer's nutritional plan. I could tell he was worried about the treatment. Clint followed every single rule from every single doctor and therapist. Clint did the same thing when the Western doctors were in charge, with imminent death results. The functional doctor's ideas were extremely slow, but they were going in the right direction.

At that point, I was not concerned about toxicologist Dr. Boshaft from ULTRA tracking down Clint. The bill for every current treatment was being paid with cash. No more insurance information was being given out. We no longer had a paper trail. It's interesting that our government insists this new electronic medical record-keeping system is "all for the good of US citizens." I still wonder if the numerous blood test results processed through insurance made their way into Dr. Boshaft's hands.

Clint was still deathly sick, but I kept learning a little more each day. I was unsure whether this was a good thing but didn't know what else to do.

Clint's schedule was very busy, as he was constantly going somewhere for a therapy appointment.

I kept working, trying to stay ahead of the bills. Both of us were just trying to stay alive, trying to keep our heads above water.

Clint's heavy-metal tests results came back. The reports said what Dr. Fritzmeyer and I already knew. Clint was, indeed, poisoned. His natural trace minerals had been replaced with heavy metals. He had a small amount of arsenic. His biggest enemy was barium.

All soluble barium compounds are poisonous to humans. This is most likely because they interfere with the functioning of potassium ion channels in the body.

Arsenic is a common n-type dopant in semiconductor electronic devices. Arsenic compounds are well absorbed within twenty-four hours and redistributed to the liver, lungs, intestinal wall, and spleen, where they bind to the sulfhydryl groups of tissue proteins. Arsenic also replaces phosphorus in the bone, where it may remain for years. Hence, the effects of chronic poisoning still can be seen years after exposure has stopped. Signs and symptoms of chronic arsenic poisoning may not occur until two to eight weeks after exposure. Clint left ULTRA at the end of July. His flu-like symptoms began in September. Yet Dr. Boshaft, the toxicologist, told Clint his illnesses could not be caused by arsenic because the effects of exposure are instantaneous. He lied.

Clint's blood tests showed high levels of arsenic. Yet his doctor was not concerned at all. As it crept into his bones, the blood and urine tests showed less and less.

Go back to the beginning of this book and read what Ultra manufactured. Read what they used to make their semiconductors. I finally had my proof. I could medically show, after all these years, that Clint was still being poisoned by barium and arsenic. It was the cause of my son's imminent death. Ultra and Dr. Boshaft knew this.

I repeat: Doping is a process by which manufacturers create semiconductors. It involves adding an impurity (e.g., barium) to a pure chemical (usually silicon) to create an imbalance in the electronic fields. This creates semiconductors.

When barium accumulates in the body, it usually affects the functions of the nervous system. Barium poisoning displays symptoms that are similar to flu, which is why it is not strange to find the condition misdiagnosed as flu. Clint's first symptom in 2004, after leaving Ultra, was stomach flu.

Signs and symptoms: Short-term exposure: Alkaline barium compounds, such as the hydroxide and carbonate, may cause local irritation to the eyes, nose, throat, and skin. Exposure to either form can affect the nervous system and cause hyperkalemia, which can cause heart disorders. Long-term exposure: Barium poisoning is virtually unknown in industry, although the potential exists when the soluble forms are used. When ingested or given orally, the soluble, ionized barium compounds exert a *profound effect on all **muscles*** and especially smooth muscles, markedly increasing their *contractility.* The heart rate is slowed and may stop in systole. Other effects are increased intestinal peristalsis, vascular constriction, *bladder contraction*, and increased *voluntary muscle tension.* The inhalation of the dust of barium sulfate may lead to deposition in the lungs in sufficient quantities to produce "baritosis" (benign pneumoconiosis). This produces a radiologic picture in the absence of symptoms and abnormal physical signs. X-rays, however, will show disseminated nodular opacities throughout the lung fields, which are discrete, but sometimes overlap.

/Alkaline barium compounds/[1]

---

[1] R. P. Pohanish, ed. *Sittig's Handbook of Toxic and Hazardous Chemical Carcinogens* (Norwich, NY: William Andrew), 293.

His other issues (see listing below) were chromium, nickel, zinc, selenium, and aluminum, with mercury close behind. Titanium and lead were tied. And the list went on. None registered in the high range. A few were in the above-normal range. Dr. Fritzmeyer said there were just too many! The other problem was that they only checked for twenty-six heavy metals. There are many more for which they didn't check.

	Result
	µg/g
Arsenic (As)	0.015
Lead (Pb)	0.14
Mercury (Hg)	0.44
Cadmium (Cd)	0.03**
Chromium (Cr)	0.41
Beryllium (Be)	< 0.01
Cobalt (Co)	0.009
Nickel (Ni)	0.18
Zinc (Zn)	180
Copper (Cu)	11
Thorium (Th)	< 0.001
Thallium (TI)	0.001
Barium (Ba)	1.8

Cesium Cs)	<0.002
Manganese (Mn)	0.15
Selenium (Se)	0.87
Bismuth (Bi)	0.013
Vanadium (V)	0.022
Silver (Ag)	0.15
Antimony (Sb)	0.87
Palladium (Pd)	0.013
Aluminum (Al)	0.022
Platinum (Pt)	<0.006
Tungsten (W)	0.002
Tin (Sn)	0.12
Uranium (U)	0.016
Gold (Au)	0.004
Tellurium (Te)	<0.05
Germanium(Ge)	0.031
Titanium (Ti)	0.26
Gadolinium(Gd)	<0.001

Are the metals mixing and making more inside of him, like a bad chemistry experiment? I wondered as I looked at the report. I'd have to look into that as well. Like learning disabilities, these metals in small amounts, by themselves, were not alarming. It was the number of them in one person's body that becomes overwhelming. Again, the percentage of metals registering in Clint's hair was no longer accurate. The metals were now permanent residents of his organs, brain, bones, and soft tissue. Most likely, the original invader would have been well above the acceptable level when Clint first became ill. I feel that since our government and medical world refuse to acknowledge heavy-metal toxicity in chronic cases, the levels of absorption are never truly measured. The body break-down begins, the metals find safe harbor, and the proof that is needed is lost. The sick person dies of over body toxicity. The doctor diagnoses an acceptable, common cause of death, and then everyone says, "What a shame; he was so young," and goes on with life.

More than ever, I needed a chemist to research what ULTRA did in Pennsylvania. I seriously needed a chemist to tie Clint's heavy-metal test result to ULTRA. I didn't have time. All of my efforts were being pushed into saving his life.

All of this research had to wait until December 2014.

Now I think I know what I needed to know in order to save my son. Hindsight is twenty/twenty. The discovery was made too late in so many different arenas, from permanent health issues, through the total interruption of life. It's too late for legal action. Clint most will likely never work again. I will never retire. It is so unfair.

I remember that it was a Wednesday, but I can't remember if it was the end of July or the middle of August. We had just finished with chamber time, and I was leaving for my Wednesday job.

We said our goodbyes, and I left, worrying about money. Clint was hurrying to the bathroom to throw up, as he did every morning. *He has morning sickness*, I thought as I climbed into my car.

I greeted everyone when I arrived at the office. The owner of Amusements Rental, Dan, came to ask me what he could do to help me. He had heard of my serious situation.

"Well, money is a serious concern. I spent $6,500 on an oxygen chamber for Clint," I explained. "And now, Clint's about to start EDTA infusion therapy at the end of the month. That costs $175 twice a week, or about a thousand dollars each month. Insurance is not an option anymore. He goes to physical therapy a couple of times a week. Unfortunately, I have no idea how long this is going to go on."

"Wow," he said sympathetically. "How long have you been battling this illness?"

"Since before I started working here," I told him. At that very moment, an idea occurred to me. "Hey! Can we do a fund-raiser? You have all the latest and greatest inflatable fun toys here. Could we possibly use them for a fund-raising event for Clint?"

The next thing I knew, Dan had put together a team for me. And not the type of team urologist Dr. Barstow would recommend, not a team of people who wear scrubs. Dan put together an A-1 winning team. And I was happy! Dan had five people, some of whom I had never before met, rushing around to help *me*. They worked and worked and worked.

Dan put the word out to all of his friends that he needed a group to help raise money for Clint. Dan's a US Marine. One might normally say an ex-marine, but as I have come to learn, "Once a marine, always a marine," and Dan certainly fit the profile. He wanted to save everyone. He asked his VA buddies from the VFW group to have a motorcycle ride fund-raiser. They said yes! His buddy Sarge volunteered to be on the committee. Another business associate and her husband, who were motorcyclists, also agreed to be on the committee. Dan's girlfriend joined the group. Before I even met the committee, the plans were set for October 1.

Dan contacted the local bar that usually hosted his fund-raising and secured the owner's agreement to host our event. October weather should be perfect.

The committee was assigned to oversee the bike-ride event. I was in charge of the secret auction, raffle prizes, and food. That meant I needed my own committee. I had no problem with that. My sisters were all in. Even my friends, whom I'd neglected, jumped in to help. Everything was rolling, and we had less than six weeks until the big day.

I began visiting merchants in my neighborhood. Everyone I stopped in to see agreed to give me something to raffle. My sisters did the same in their communities. Two of my friends who work for Proctor and Gamble filled baskets with P&G products. Dan put together the grand prize of a scooter cooler filled with adult drinks. It was the big money-maker. We had more than thirty silent auction prizes and many raffle prizes as well.

Then I gathered volunteers to bring the food. Many people cooked savory dishes and baked goodies. Dan donated the money that the other volunteers used to shop for the paper products and picnic condiments. It was going to be one fabulous event!

On the last Wednesday in September, it was sixty-five degrees and a fabulous fall day. On the Friday before the event, I began simmering my homemade bean soup. It kept growing and growing into additional huge pots as the day turned into night. As I was cooking, the sky filled with clouds. The temperature dropped by twenty degrees. Rain poured down. It turned into winter overnight, and by Saturday morning, it was frosty cold.

Bike riders didn't show to ride, of course. It was simply too cold and dangerous. In spite of the disappointment, the volunteers kept up their spirits.

It was so cold that we held the auction and raffle inside the bar. The food, music, and party was supposed to be outside. Dan had set up his mechanical bull down in the parking lot. Bull rides were two dollars. The bar owner agreed to donate the soft drinks and give the five-dollar cover charge to the cause. We were all set—except for the weather.

Many people came to this event. The committee invited many of their friends and family to attend. High school friends of Clint's and his brother's came. My friends and their families and many of my clients came. Despite the disappointing weather, it turned out to be an exceptional party. We raised a little over ten thousand dollars, thanks to Dan. The fund-raiser was a great success, thanks to generous clients, great friends, supportive family, and people I didn't even know.

Clint felt well enough to come to the event for a few hours. I think the event itself helped Clint's spirits more than the money that we raised.

The next thank-you went to Clint's uncle. He took charge and talked with Grams. Remember Grams, the grandma in Alabama that Clint went to see before coming home in April 2010? Clint's uncle asked if she would convert some of her future "will money" to help Clint. He helped set up a medical trust fund that paid for all of the EDTA infusions. Many thanks to Grams.

With the money problem somewhat under control, Clint could concentrate on getting well.

Functional medicine is a patient-centered healing process. Rather than looking at each symptom as a separate issue, the doctor realizes that the patient's body is no longer in balance. Functional medicine first identifies the reasons for this imbalance. Then the symptoms are treated in a way that the body can heal itself. This type of patient treatment allows each person to be treated according to his or her personal health needs, instead of a one-pill-fixes-all treatment approach. In reality, the one pill creates more imbalances, while covering up the root of the illnesses, causing it to worsen while creating more disease.

September 2011

I called my oldest sister on September 1. "Hi, Laura," I said. "Clint needs to get to Lewisburg, and his hips are causing him so much pain I'm afraid that he won't make it, riding in my car with bucket seats. He's still really sick. Can I borrow your van?"

"Of course you can," she said.

Everyone in my family wanted to help. Everyone was pulling for Clint.

Two months after the latest AVN decompression on September 7, Clint had to get into the car and ride over ninety minutes to visit with a toxicologist.

Dr. Boshaft's threat had proven real. I felt ULTRA's power. He had shut us down in Charleston. But I believed I had outsmarted him by going to Lewisburg. The Chicago and Dallas incident didn't seem real enough to think that Dr. Boshaft would go that far to stop Clint from getting well. I chalked it up to coincidence.

Clint was throwing up the day we had to leave, but he pulled it together. "Come on; let's go," he said, still a little green.

I started the van, and Clint climbed into the back seat to lie down. I looked in the rearview mirror and just wanted to cry. *Why is this happening? What happens if I am wrong? What happens if he's sick for some other reason than the one I think? I'm not a doctor. Who am I to decide that he's sick because of chemical poisoning?* With effort, I shook the thoughts from my head. *Stay the course. Stick with your gut. Remember the unrelated multiple symptoms that just don't connect. He is poisoned.*

I backed the car down the drive and pulled away. In the rearview mirror, I could see Clint gritting his teeth in pain. *Please let this day bring what we need,* I prayed.

I drove to Lewisburg. Clint tried to sleep on the way. In an hour and a half, we arrived at the Medical Toxicology Department of West Virginia Health with high hopes.

Clint crawled out of the back seat. "Let's just get through this day," he said, grabbing for his crutches. We slowly walked to the office, per the instructions we had received in the mail. All the paperwork was filled out.

As we entered the door to Dr. Roget's office, my heart pounded strongly in a chest that was suddenly squeezed too tightly. *Ba-boom! Ba-boom! Ba-boom!* My heart pounded, as it always did when I was about face a potentially arrogant doctor.

Think happy thoughts, I told myself. *She said she was the best in the area. She said she would be able to help. It's going to happen. She's going to detoxify Clint from these horrible monsters that are eating him alive.*

"I'm here to see Dr. Roget," Clint said after introducing himself.

As Clint signed in, the receptionists looked up in confusion. "Who are you?"

"Oh no," I murmured.

Clint and the woman conversed another moment; then she made a phone call to find out why Clint's name was not on the appointment list, and his records were not in the new-patient file on her desk.

I was starting to perspire, and my stomach churned in fear. Clint couldn't take another day like this! But what choice did we have?

The receptionist finished her phone conversation and turned to Clint with a small, tight smile. "You need to go to the second floor," she said with a slight nod. "Dr. Roget is going to see you there, rather than here with her normal patients."

I could see in his face that this scared Clint. We went back down to the second floor and sat silently in the waiting room. We had no idea what department was housed there. We were in a waiting room that looked just like any other.

"Clint? Clint Marshall?" we heard a voice call from the door at the end of the room. Clint stood, wincing in pain as he grabbed for his crutches. I followed him into the examination room, carrying the jam-packed three-ring binder. I had urine test results and hair tests that showed heavy metals. I had Dr. Fritzmeyer's information that confirmed what I thought. I had many records that contained critical information.

Dr. Roget finally joined us in the examination room. She was maybe twenty-seven years old, certainly no more than thirty. *Where's all this*

learned experience that she claimed to have when I made this appointment?
I wondered.

"Hello," she said. "My name is Dr. Roget. I am a neurotoxicologist." She
began to examine Clint. She had him stick out his tongue. She had him
push down on her hands. She held up one finger and moved it in front of
his eyes. She did the usual stuff, nothing exceptional.

"You are not poisoned," she said authoritatively. "You don't have
metal toxicity or over body burden." My head began to spin. I felt like I
was slipping into a hole in the ground. "You have too many unrelated
symptoms, which I believe are related to a mental disorder. I recommend
that you seek help from a psychiatrist. Your pain is caused by a
depression and anxiety disorder."

"Excuse me?" Clint said. "What caused my hips to die, then? Why do I
have arthritis? What is causing my joints to lock in place? Why am I sick
all the time? Why do my hair and urine tests keep coming back containing
metals?"

The room seemed to darken. My mouth was dry, and I couldn't
breathe, let alone speak. *What is happening to me? Talk,* I told myself. But I
couldn't. I was frozen.

Dr. Roget took a deep breath and, seeming to select her words
carefully, said, "Everyone has metals. It's just the world we live in. Your
amounts are so low that they couldn't be causing you all these problems.
Yours are typical symptoms associated with depression."

I was in utter and complete shock.

"How did the metals get there?" Clint asked. "Where did the titanium,
barium, selenium, germanium, and arsenic come from? The lead is clearly
out of accepted levels."

Dr. Roget was ready for that question. "You get metals from the air,
from your shampoo, from your water. Do you drink the tap water in your
house? Charleston has bad water, you know. You are not sick from your
job. If you had been poisoned by arsine gas in 2004, your kidneys would

have shut down, and you would be dead or, at the very least, have cancer by now. You need to accept the fact that this is *not* heavy-metal-related. You need to go on antidepressants and find a pain-management doctor. I'm sorry, but I can't help you."

Wait, I thought. *This sounds like the Dr. Boshaft speech. Some of her sentences are close to the ones that Dr. Boshaft uttered last July.*

Clint smirked at Dr. Roget. "Well, I am going to go buy every single bottle of Herbal Essence shampoo I can find. I'm going to stand on my front porch twenty-four/seven and collect more gold and nickel in my hair. I'm going to breathe in real deep and fill my lungs with all kinds of precious metals so when I die, my mom can recycle my body to pay your bill."

Dr. Roget turned quickly. Looking at her, I saw a little nervous line around her mouth. She was twitchy, jittery. She had the same look that Dr. Khanna would get when something violated his comfort zone.

Finding my voice, I said, "You are a neurologist, right? You have the ability to test Clint to see what's neurologically wrong. Can't you? Can we back up and move in that direction? Maybe we are missing something in the brain." I took a deep breath, trying to focus. "You haven't even looked at my book." I hated the pleading tone in my voice, yet I was unable to prevent it. I held out the binder, offering it to her. "I want to ask you questions about some of these tests. I need your expert opinion as to why some of these tests say what they do. Can you please look at the hormone tests? Please look at the tissue mineral tests. I know you'll be able to read them and know why his levels are so out of balance."

"No," Dr. Roget answered quickly. "I can't see him anymore. You need to stay in Charleston, close to home. Find a physiatrist near your home and get some help with your mental issues. I'll write a lab order to have Clint's blood tested for arsenic. Will that make you feel better?"

I knew the arsenic had been testing very low in Clint's hair tests. Dr. Fritzmeyer already told me that the metals in Clint's blood had moved deep into his tissues and brain, so testing for the metals was pretty much a waste of time. The only way to find out what was in his bones was by getting a *bone* sample. The time to test his blood had long passed. *And those bones are gone,* I thought.

Dr. Roget handed Clint a blood-drawing prescription and briskly left the room.

Feeling numb, Clint and I went downstairs to have his blood taken. We both knew she would prove herself right about the absence of arsenic in his blood at this time.

"I am just going to die. You can't save me. I am just going to die," Clint said miserably.

My mind raced. *What am I missing? What is going on?* We stopped for dinner on the way home. Clint had another negative day to overcome, and I had another medical bill to pay.

When we got home, I decided to see if ULTRA had an office in Lewisburg. Bingo—it was on 746 North Highland Road, about fifteen miles from the Baptist hospital. I knew she sounded like Dr. Boshaft. I began to wonder if her school loans had just been paid off with the money she must have received in return for lying to us.

Clint called the number on our West Virginia Health paperwork to talk to the medical team there. We needed copies of the prior day's visit for my binder.

"I was there yesterday and had an appointment with Dr. Roget. I need a copy of the report regarding my visit," he said.

"One moment, please. What's your name again? I don't have your information in the computer. What is your Social? Are you sure it was in this office?"

"Yes, I was there, seeing Dr. Roget. This is her office, yes?"

"Yes, it is, but your name is not on her patient list. Can you hang on a minute?" She put him on hold for about five minutes. "I had to call downstairs to see if they had your paperwork. It's really strange. We can't find your information anywhere."

"What do you mean? What? Like I was never there?" Clint cried, incredulous and angry. "Has this ever happened before?"

"No, I can't say that it ever has," she said. "Let me see if I can find your records, and I'll call you back."

A couple of hours later, Clint heard back from her. "I finally found your records. The file was buried in a drawer in Dr. Roget's office—very strange! Well, at least I found it. We're getting to the bottom of this. Thanks for the phone call. Your file would have been lost forever."

I knew that Dr. Boshaft was in the middle of all of this. His threats kept repeating in my mind. Researching Dr. Boshaft, I found quite a bit of information. It seemed that he was a big shot. He ran the toxicology department at CAMC (Charleston Area Medical Center), the very place we had tried to access in the spring. He was the gatekeeper! He also sat on the board at Saint Clair's. He had access to all of Clint's medical records. All he needed to do was go into the system and look up Clint's name. I think he already had his Social Security number from the emergency room visit. *Am I beginning to learn what I need to learn in order to figure out what I need to know—or am I just going crazy?* I wondered. *I think I'm on to something here.*

Dr. Boshaft was the consulting physician for ULTRA the entire time they were in Pennsylvania. ULTRA had an ambulance and helicopter on site, right there in Cranberry Township. ULTRA seemed to be everywhere and to have their hands in everything. When people were injured at the ULTRA plant, they were flown to CAMC or Saint Clair—and Dr. Boshaft was their physician.

"That's the last straw," I said. We wouldn't be using insurance ever again. No more insurance card. No more feeding Dr. Boshaft information! If he *was* behind this confrontation with Dr. Roget, he knew what we were doing before we did. Could he look up Clint through the new medical record system that the government had just designed and track Clint's every move? Now Dr. Boshaft had a sample of Clint's blood. Most likely, he had all of Clint's records that I, in good faith, had sent to Dr. Roget. HIPAA regulations—what a joke!

For the next few days, Clint spent his time calling Herbal Essences, asking if they knew that heavy metals were in their shampoo. They were not very happy about Dr. Roget's accusing them of making Clint sick. Herbal Essences promised Clint that their shampoo *did not* contain heavy metals. Clint called the Greater Charleston Water Works. They also were very unhappy that Dr. Roget accused them of having arsenic, barium, and germanium in their water. They told Clint they planned to send the water-testing reports to prove that the water was not poisonous.

Busy developing the next idea, I forgot to watch for the records that Clint had requested the day after the appointment. It was no surprise that the report from Dr. Roget never showed up. That record is lost forever. I figure it was burned. The report was never sent to Dr. Tiens, as Dr. Roget promised she would do on the day of our appointment. Dr. Tiens called several times and requested it. It never arrived. I wonder if the blood sample was really tested for arsenic or frozen and put into a vault someplace as a just-in-case need for Dr. Boshaft.

October 2011

"How are you feeling?" I asked Clint after his first day of EDTA.

"Not so good," he answered. He looked dead. His skin was gray, and his face was etched in pain.

"It will get better," I assured him, hoping it was true.

Clint and I moved into a holding pattern. He continued to see Tim to work on his hips. He went for his EDTA infusions twice a week. They were really hard on him.

I got the feeling that Dr. Fritzmeyer did not approve of the EDTA treatments, but he kept a positive position with his nutritional treatment plan.

Dr. Tiens gave Clint glutathione intravenously before each EDTA infusion and sold Clint a canister of supplements that he wanted him to take along with the supplements Dr. Fritzmeyer had given him. They were called BC chelation.

November 2011

The EDTA infusions stirred things up within Clint. His skin broke out in rashes, and, at times, he looked especially jaundiced. His teeth shone with a silver translucent glow. His bladder was worse than ever.

Dr. Fritzmeyer had told us during that first visit, "Detoxification is an extremely painful process. Every pain and symptom that you have had in the past eight years will rear its ugly head. Pain will leave your body in the opposite order that the symptoms appeared. Most likely, since the urinary issue was the first and worst and still hanging on, it will be the last to leave and the worst throughout this process. The general rule of thumb is however many years you have been poisoned is how many years it will take to get detoxified."

"Clint," I said to him one night after a treatment. "I'm worried. What is going on? You look awful."

"Look!" he snapped. "You think I look bad? You should feel how I feel. This EDTA stuff has got something happening inside of me. I have no idea if that's good or bad. The holes that Dr. Khanna drilled in my legs feel really funny."

"What do you mean, funny?" I asked.

"I swear I can feel something coming out of them. Like a dull ache and then some pulses. It's hard to explain. It's weird. There's a dull ache, and then pain travels down my leg, into my knee, into my ankle, and out the bottom of my foot!"

Clint continued to go to Dr. Tiens for his EDTA infusions, no matter how he was feeling. Good or bad, he kept on going. He would be throwing up as he walked out the door. He still went.

Early in December, he turned to me. "It may be too early to say this—and I hope I don't jinx myself—but I think it's working."

Oh my God! For the first time in two years, my son said something positive about his condition! I glimpsed a ray of hope, a small stroke of sunlight coming our way.

Tim was helping with his hip strength, in spite of Dr. Khanna, and Dr. Tiens was working on the EDTA infusions.

One day, Clint walked upstairs after an EDTA infusion. "Hey, look at this!" he exclaimed, pointing at the inside of his elbow. He had developed a lump about three inches wide. It had swelled up to about the size of a tangerine. The skin was stretched and had an oily discharge.

"This is new," he said. With each EDTA infusion, his symptoms got more unusual. Dr. Tiens offered no explanation for the symptoms. He just kept telling Clint to keep up the good work.

Sometimes, after an EDTA infusion, he would get quite sick. It reminded me of seeing someone go through chemotherapy.

Here we go again, I thought. "Just the two of us," I sang the jazz classic, trying to make him laugh. "We can make it if we try. Just the two of us, you and I!"

We were all alone, trying to figure out what to do. Clint needed more help. As the toxins began to move, his soft tissue pain intensified.

Clint decided to talk to Dr. Tiens about it. "My muscles are twitching more since we started this process. I hurt all over. My mom says I need deep-tissue massages to help get the trapped poisons out through my skin. She read about it on the internet. There's a special technique to it; it's not just a massage. I need someone that will twist out the poison that is trapped."

This technique is used on fibromyalgia sufferers. I believe

fibromyalgia is caused by heavy metals, and the Western medical world is not allowed to say that. I also believe pelvic-floor disease and endometriosis are, in some cases, caused by heavy-metal over body burden. Furthermore, Lyme disease is not what we think it is. Rather, I believe the medical conditions that follow after a person is treated for a deer-tick bite come from the metals that are in the antidote injections. I have had many email conversations with people who have been diagnosed with Lyme disease. Could the drugs that they are given, which contain metals in order to stay in the brain, be causing symptoms similar to Clint's and be the real reason for their life sentence of pain? Or could it be from the high doses of antibiotics that are prescribed? Or do their bodies simply go out of balance due to the tick's venom. Maybe all these people need is a body-out-of-balance adjustment. Since that treatment plan would not include Big Pharma drugs, it will never be accepted by the Western medical world.

Dr. Tiens considered the deep-tissue massage therapy. "That's a really great idea. There is a woman named Meg in this building who does some deep-tissue massage therapies. Let's talk with her."

Meg was another one of the "good guys" I kept adding to my team. She kept detailed notes of every visit Clint ever had. She truly cared. Clint could call her cell phone, any day, any time, and she would always answer. She researched and leaned new techniques to help relieve Clint's pain. When I told her that I wanted to write a book, and asked her to be part of it, she sent the following email message to me:

> When I first met Clint, he slowly walked down the hall. I could see his labored walking. I would not describe this as a far walk, but for him it was. One of the first things I noticed was how tired and worn out his young body appeared. The color of Clint's skin was light gray, and the odor that came from his body was very foul. His muscles

had atrophied, and he was so thin I wondered how a person that young could have such unhealthy conditions. I was more than concerned.

Clint had been referred to me for massage therapy by a doctor in the same building. I listened as Clint told me what I know now was only a very small portion of his story about his health. He had lived with constant pain, like knives in his flesh. He had endured hip surgeries, the feeling of being strangled, the swelling of his lymph nodes, and severe lack of sleep. He was so tired it was overwhelming. Many specialists and doctors had dismissed his concerns. He was hesitant to add another failed therapy attempt to his collection.

But what Clint found was me—a person who listened to his words and his body. Each visit he opened up a little more until I heard the whole story. I would listen and then massage his body, finding multiple areas of adhesions, trigger points, and the knots that needed to be broken down, hoping to release the trapped toxins. I trailed to wherever it led me. Each visit was different. I constantly worked his body, never certain where those visits would lead. There were many times when I questioned my work: was I able to help him? Seeing Clint each visit showed me that it was working.

Clint would do whatever it took to get better: swimming, stretching, working out, taking all the supplements, the list goes on. He kept fighting for his life. Along with all his nutrition and supplements, this holistic approach, what Clint would sometimes teasingly call voodoo, he was thriving. His skin tone returned to a healthy color. Slowly, he rebuilt his once-frail body—and now he is muscular once more.

Of course, there are still the times when he slides back. That's when I'll get the call to schedule his massage treatment. But to have outlived his doctors' diagnoses of certain death is huge!

His mom, Peggy, has been his lifeline. Without her support and digging through mountains of research, I don't think Clint would be here today. She was determined to find an answer to this madness and support her son no matter what.

From seeing Clint two times a week since 2011, it's very rare to see him these days. To me, that's great; it tells me that he is living! I am quite happy to know this can be overcome. I'm very happy to be part of his story of returning to good health.

I am so glad to see Clint living again!

Yes, you may freely use my name and location.

—Meg Masters, [INSIDE ADDRESS], URL for Meg Masters Massage

Next, I'd like to share with you my email message to Dr. Tiens and Nurse Roberta on the eve of Thanksgiving 2011.

Dear Dr. Tiens and Nurse Roberta,

It's Thanksgiving and I am choosing you to be my Thanksgiving tribute for this year. Clint has only been coming to see you since August. Because of your gentle care and courage to try the impossible, Clint seems to be feeling a little better. Thank you very much for being there for him and me. You are the best.

They sent me a thank-you email message the next day, apologizing for taking so long to respond to my Thanksgiving email. Dr. Tiens and Nurse Roberta had been out the entire night, sitting with an elderly woman who was dying. She had been their patient for a very long time. This was Dr. Tiens's and Nurse Roberta's life—taking care of others. I knew that Clint and I had found our angels.

December 2011

"Happy birthday," I said on the morning of December 12, Clint's thirty-sixth birthday. "How did you sleep? Are you feeling any better?"

Why do I ask? I wondered. *Why do I insist on asking the question, knowing that I will not want to hear the answer? He has been sick for almost eight years. Many doctors have said that he* should *be dead. But here he is, waiting to climb into the chamber: his own little tunnel of hell. He barely fits inside. With his auditory disability, the noises that echo in from the outside world are multiplied. The compressor that keeps the tube under pressure hisses. It's his birthday, and he's going into his own little version of hell because this sickness doesn't take a day off, not even on his birthday.*

The window in the chamber had lost its inner seal, and there were air bubbles between the two sheets of plastic. Clint could no longer look at me through it. He couldn't hear inside the chamber, and now he couldn't read my lips either. The chamber had become a source of contention.

"Clint, it's your birthday. If you want to take the day off from the chamber, it is okay," I offered.

"No way," he said. "It's working. I'm feeling better." He was feeling better only during *some* parts of an hour. "I don't want my hips to die. I cannot or *will not* go through anything like that again. I need my hips. I'm going back to work."

"Happy birthday," I said again. "Climb on in."

Clint worked his way through the rest of December, one day at a time. He was beginning to look better than he had looked in a very long time.

It was Christmas Day, and Clint was finally looking at least half alive.

"Merry Christmas," I said. Clint grinned, and I knew what he was thinking. Most days were still painful. But some hours weren't all that bad. We'd take it.

In spite of the progress he was making, his sister, Sarah, came into town for Christmas, deeply concerned that it might be Clint's last.

Thirteen

More Good People (2012)

January 2012

I decided to go with Clint to see Dr. Tiens. Clint was improving, and I wanted to hear what he thought. I greeted him as we entered his office, and he welcomed us with a warm smile.

"I didn't think it could be done. I really didn't expect his liver to be saved. He did it!"

"No," I said. "You and Nurse Roberta did it. We were just along for the ride."

Clint continued to get the EDTA infusions. The veins in his arms were becoming fibrous. As the infusion therapy drew to an end, Clint and I realized that the EDTA was not in him long enough to grab hold of the poison way down deep inside his tissues and bones. EDTA could easily grab the metals in the blood. Chelation therapy was coming to an end.

I researched EDTA to find out how long it stays in a person's blood. It turns out it is only a few hours and therefore can only attach to the metals that are easily accessed. I read that our military hospitals treat some special war heroes with EDTA in secret medical facilities. The men go into the facilities undercover for a couple of days. They just disappear. Their blood is run through a detoxification process for twenty-four hours straight. Only a few people are given that privilege and have to fight for it. Regular hardworking people like my son are left to die. Such a death is usually given an accepted death reason and quickly forgotten by physicians who, I believe, are not allowed to speak the truth.

February 2012

Clint went backward. The urinary issues, along with all the rest of his symptoms, seemed to be coming back. "Mom," Clint said. "I'm sick again. I feel like I did last fall."

I was very worried. *Now what?*

Back in heavy research mode, I scanned through pages and pages of internet advertisements touting supplement after supplement as the answer to removing heavy metals.

"Mom," Clint called to me. "Look up DMSA. I heard about DMSA versus EDTA therapy today."

"I'm on it!" Looking it up, I found that Meso-2,3-dimercaptosuccinic acid (DMSA) is a compound, approved in the 1960s by the FDA, for the removal (chelation) of heavy metals. Liking what I read about its efficacy, I ordered the supplements for Clint.

He mixed and matched supplements and vitamins to find out which combinations helped him feel the best. Dr. Fritzmeyer's nutritional plan was still intact. Clint followed it like his bible. Dr. Fritzmeyer didn't entirely trust DMSA and said that it could cause more harm than good.

Eventually, Clint decided to jump fully on the DMSA bandwagon anyway.

Clint decided while taking DMSA that there was a lot to consider. EDTA and DMSA both act like magnets for metals. Instead of an infusion, DMSA is a pill. Because it's a pill, Clint could take it all day long. He could take twenty-five milligrams or a hundred milligrams or a combination of the two. The EDTA with Dr. Tiens was about to end. We needed to figure out something else, and Dr. Tiens only knew EDTA.

Clint learned that DMSA pulled the metals out—great. It would remove trace minerals and the heavy metals that mimic trace minerals. The heavy metals have to be neutralized in order to sneak by the liver and intestines. If he took too much DMSA, he could retoxify the liver. If he did that too many times, the liver could become overburdened. The cleansing process would stop, and the poisons would once again take over. His liver would begin to die again.

The next most important ingredients that a person has to have are amino and alpha lipoic acids—protein. These protein acids attach to the metals and allow them to pass through the liver and escape through the intestines. It was a chemistry lesson that I decided was true. I'm really not sure if it works that way, but it seemed like it while we were doing it.

Clint and I were not chemists, so we had to learn the hard way. Clint understood that the DMSA was removing everything: the good, the bad, and the ugly. A few hours after taking the DMSA, he started to take trace minerals and his other supplements, with the goal of pulling out the bad and then pushing in the good.

In this process, working up a good sweat was extremely important. No matter how sick Clint was, he never spent his days in bed, curled up in a ball, as he had in previous years. He now knew that he needed to work the muscles to release the toxins. Let the DMSA attach to them. Drink a lot of water. He knew not to eat sugar and to eat healthy food. He knew to take protein acids and sweat. That was the plan. All the while, the good stuff had to be replaced. Clint began light workouts to sweat out the poisons.

Clint was following Dr. Fritzmeyer's plan, and he incorporated his own ideas. He also continued to see Dr. Tiens for his EDTA. We felt that the DMSA was digging deeply into his bones and tissues. On the EDTA days, his liver was getting help with the glutathione infusions while the EDTA grabbed the heavy metals that were being forced out of the bones and into his bloodstream, with the help from the DMSA on the other days.

Honestly, we had no definitive idea. But it's what we believed. What we do know is that it helped. Clint was still feeling sick much of the time. His hips were still in constant pain. Every day, we worried that something else was wrong.

"Mom," Clint called for me in a panic. "I think I need to have an MRI of my hips. I need to know that everything is okay." His hips had been aching more than usual. We didn't have an orthopedic doctor anymore because Lighthouse Orthopedic refused to return our calls or make any appointments concerning Clint's hips. New orthopedic doctors that we did see refused to accept him as a new patient. They didn't want to take on that liability. Clint was a man without a doctor. All said the decompression surgery would never work, and soon Clint would need hip replacements.

"Call the MRI center and see what the going rate is for an out-of-pocket MRI," I told him. I had given up a long time ago trying to convince the insurance companies that we needed MRIs of Clint's hips.

Necrosis is not well understood. The only way to know if the hips have AVN is to have an MRI, so I paid for them and chose when we would go.

Clint called Dr. Khanna and requested an appointment and an MRI referral. Dr. Khanna's personal assistant began to rant about how difficult it would to get the insurance company to pay for an MRI. She told him that he was discharged, and the hips were no longer Dr. Khanna's responsibility. Clint argued. She asked Clint to hang on for a minute. She came back to the phone with a huge sigh and agreed to make him one final appointment.

"I'll pay for them myself. Let's just skip the insurance. I need to know where I am," Clint told her. Lighthouse knew that; he was not a new patient.

My parents had sent a check in the mail. *Why do people always somehow know when I really need cash?* I didn't talk too much to anyone about what we were doing. No one seemed to understand what was happening, and constantly explaining had become exhausting. It took too much time, and people got overwhelmed when I tried. The check paid for the MRI. I was profoundly grateful.

March 2012

MRI results in hand, we went to see Dr. Khanna, even though he was becoming more useless every time we showed up. He was guarded and would not give us direct answers. Perhaps he thought that I might sue because necrosis can be caused by hip dislocations.

I knew that Dr. Savvin did not cause the AVN, and I knew that Drs. Savvin and Khanna saved my son's hips and legs. I would never sue them. None of this was their fault. But I couldn't give up my game face. I am a warrior.

Clint was concerned that the DMSA and EDTA were hurting his hips. He was afraid that the AVN was coming back. The pain in his hips was not the same as it was in 2011. Understandably, the idea of losing his hips and legs was extremely scary. He had to know.

"Why are you here? Who told you to come in?" Dr. Khanna asked. This seemed so strange, as the protocol for AVN was an annual checkup for the next five years.

"I want to be sure my hips are healing okay. It has been more than nine months, and I'm worried." We didn't even try to tell Dr. Khanna about Clint's detoxification process.

When he had examined the MRI and the just-taken x-ray, Dr. Khanna smiled broadly. "Your hips are beautiful," he said. "The drill holes are all filled in and as white as can be. You do still have a spot of AVN on the left side. We'll have to watch that. It may still regenerate to 100 percent as the red blood cells repair the damage. Keep up the good work.

I thought, *We have to watch this? We can't even make an appointment without a fight. Who's watching what?* My thoughts were loud in my head, and I was angry.

"Whatever you are doing, keep it up," he said.

I wish you would listen to us, I thought.

"When can I run, jump, and play basketball?" Clint asked.

"Why would you ever want to do that?" Dr. Khanna asked.

"Do you think I will ever be able to go back to work?" Clint shot back.

Dr. Khanna reminded Clint of the conversation they'd had last May. "Not in the construction world. You're going to have to find an office job."

"I still can't work. My hips hurt all day long. If I sit, I hurt. If I stand, I hurt. Can you please help me get approved for disability?"

"Lighthouse makes people able. Lighthouse doesn't make people disabled," Dr. Khanna said. This was not the first time he had said this. It's stupid, but apparently it's his motto. He threatened that if we sent him disability paperwork, he would throw it into the trash. He would not help Clint get Social Security disability income. Neither would he help Clint rehabilitate his hips. *Why not?*

Without a doctor to admit what Clint had been through or predict his future in regard to his health, Clint couldn't get disability income. For some reason, Lighthouse wouldn't help. I suspected it was because they were afraid of a lawsuit. If they said Clint was disabled, would that mean I could sue for malpractice? I thought about that for a while, and then I had to move on. I am a warrior who chooses her battles very carefully.

Clint's hips were healing. Although it was slow, they were healing. That's really all that mattered. The decompression protocol for aftercare was hip examinations every six months, with MRI screens annually. When Clint called for follow-up visits, Dr. Khanna would not see him. He told Clint he was completely healed and discharged from his care. He would no longer see him for necrosis follow-ups. Why? It was not even a year postsurgery. Something was really wrong.

Dr. Tiens agreed to help Clint qualify for disability. He knew the chances of Clint's going back to work were very slim. He filled out the paperwork regarding his general health and chemical poisoning. He admitted to the fact that he was giving him EDTA for heavy-metal detoxification.

All through the years that Clint had been sick, I had spent a lot of time in natural health food stores. I would talk to people while I shopped. I talked to the sales staff and whoever else was there to dig for ideas to ease my son's ailments.

At this point, I needed to know why Clint couldn't eat. He was hungry all the time. He just couldn't get food to go down and stay there. I needed ideas.

I stopped at the Mayfair Natural Food Store and talked with the owner, Glenn.

"Try some miso soup," he suggested. "The Eden Certified Organic brand seems to be the best that we carry. Take an organic beef marrow bone and simmer it in the miso paste with purified water. You can add cilantro and garlic to make it a detoxifying soup. It will balance his stomach. He'll be able to digest his food about fifteen minutes after he eats it. Tell him to drink a little bit about fifteen minutes before every meal. You'll be surprised at the results."

"Thanks a lot," I said before heading to the checkout stand. I was ready to start my next chemistry experiment.

When I got home, I discussed the idea with Clint. "I have a new idea to try to settle your stomach," I told him as I climbed the basement steps. "Glenn from Mayfair Natural Food Store says this will work. I'm going to mix some up, and you can try it tonight. He says the metals have made your stomach acids out of balance. He says this will do something. If it works, I don't care what it does. I will buy stock in the company!"

I mixed the soup for Clint the way the store owner told me. Clint finished his soup as quickly as I gave it to him. "Mom," Clint said with a gulp after he swallowed his last spoonful. "I'm hungry. I need dinner." I turned and looked at him. He was sitting at the counter with a grin on his face. I had a good feeling about this.

From that night on, Clint was able to eat again. I kept miso soup in the refrigerator going forward. I added carrots, celery, and brussels sprout leaves for added nutrition. All of my chatting with people had paid off. Later, I discovered that I should have been making bone broth soup and adding fermented vegetables with detoxifying spices. This proves once again that these past years have been a learning-as-I-go process.

April 2012

Clint needed more help with his hip rehabilitation. I got back on the computer to see if I could buy a reformer. A reformer is a Pilates machine designed for people like Clint, people with injuries that need rehabilitation. I discovered that I could buy my own reformer. At Lighthouse's recommendation, I had bought Clint a spinning bike in the fall of 2011, but his hips weren't strong enough for it. Riding the bike caused more pain in his hips and back.

It had been clear for a while that we needed to rethink his hip therapy—and as Dr. Khanna wasn't interested in helping, as usual, it was up to us. Dr. Khanna had said he had never heard of a reformer and had no idea how it would rehab his hips.

Surgeons only know one thing: surgery. Repairing the resultant damage is not in their wheelhouse. Supremely arrogant, they refuse to listen to their patients. If the patient is such a loser that he or she doesn't get better on his or her own, the doctor labels the patient "difficult and refusing to follow protocol." However, the surgeon never takes the time or interest to examine his protocol to see if it fits the patient's needs! The post-op patient is just pushed away, unless, of course, that patient can medically qualify for another surgery.

When I'd finally stopped to think about the hip challenges, I realized that Clint was going to have to rebuild his hips without standing on them. Standing only made the hips worse, but most rehabilitation therapies required him to stand.

The reformer, with its bedlike frame with a wheeled, moving carriage (flat platform) on it, was the answer for him. It arrived within the week. Clint could lie down, stretch, and rebuild hip strength without his body weight crushing down his spine into his disabled hips.

I sent an email message to Kit, a personal trainer and the owner of a gym five minutes from our house. When I used to have time to work out, Kit ran the spinning classes and was my Pilates trainer for more than a year. She agreed to rebuild Clint's hips. More than just a personal trainer, she had been a surgical orthopedic hip nurse for years.

Why didn't I think of this last summer? I wondered. Sometimes things happen for a reason. *Maybe Clint wasn't ready then, but he's ready to step it up in the here and now.*

I added Kit to my Good People List.

Clint started going to Haven Rehabilitation Center sometime that same year. Tim, the physical therapist at Dr. Tiens's, ran out of tricks to pull from his gym bag. Clint needed more help strengthening his hips. Once again, I had to find a new place for Clint to go. Haven Rehab had a warm water pool and knew how to help Clint. Mostly, they worked with senior citizens.

Dr. Savvin had said a few years back that Clint's hips were in worse shape than most sixty-year-olds. I decided Clint needed to go to Haven Rehab. As Clint had the hips of a senior citizen, perhaps he needed to rehabilitate like a senior citizen.

Dr. Khanna wouldn't send any paperwork to the center or return any of their phone calls. He did send the prescription giving Haven permission to work with Clint but didn't give any further help.

Clint's hips improved at a much faster pace. I happily added these people to my Good People list.

Things with Dr. Tiens's office begin to deteriorate. Nurse Roberta had a few accidents. She fell and hurt her arm. Her face was bruised a few weeks later. There were other incidents. She told me that her mom's health was failing, and it had become difficult to manage all of her responsibilities. Things continued to go downhill. Clint would go to their office for his appointments, but she didn't show up.

Clint called me after one of those missed appointments. "Nurse Roberta didn't come in again. I sat on that hard chair for over two hours, waiting. Something is really wrong here."

"Well, Clint, I guess you have to go home." I didn't know what else to say.

Dr. Tiens's office manager (also Marcel's sister) left and moved to Florida. The new girl in the office looked like she was twelve years old and acted like a spoiled brat. When Clint called the office, she answered the phone like his call was an annoyance. The office was a chaotic mess. Clint needed Dr. Tiens.

Clint wasn't much better. The most success he had found was with mixing his own supplements. He was improving, albeit slowly. It was like riding a slow-moving roller coaster—a long, laborious climb to the top, a quick breath of fresh air, and a faster, scary drop to the bottom. That was Clint's life—a slow-moving roller coaster that never really stopped because the moment we got off, we'd have to circle around and get right back on again. Clint's wellness program hung in limbo for a while, just waiting to see if he could back bend far enough to get under the lowest day to be able to rise to a higher level of living. *How low can he go?* I used to think.

May 2012

The application for disability benefits was still moving forward. Dr. Tiens recognized Clint's critical situation and his need to take the time to recover. As Clint was living life after death, Dr. Tiens did not know if he would ever fully recover.

The reason Social Security kept declining Clint's application for disability income was Dr. Khanna's refusal to fill out the required paperwork. The court even issued a subpoena, ordering to him to show up for the hearing. Dr. Fritzmeyer, Clint's nutritionist, wrote a note to take with us to the hearing regarding Clint's precarious heath situation, but Dr. Khanna didn't show up, so nothing happened.

Last fall, after Lighthouse had made it very clear that they would never ever fill out the disability paperwork, Dr. Tiens did. Dr. Khanna told us in the very beginning, "I do not fill out disability paperwork. If that paperwork comes here, this is where it goes. Straight into the garbage can, dismissed and forgotten. Doctors do not have to fill out those forms if they don't want to. I don't want to, and I will not."

Yet in their office were notices of the cost for them to fill out disability paperwork. Lighthouse lied to us. Why?

"Mom!" Clint boomed after coming home from another disappointing appointment with Nurse Roberta. "Do you think Dr. Tiens is in trouble because of me? Do you think when he filled out the Social Security paperwork and admitted to giving me the EDTA infusions for the purpose of heavy-metal detoxification, someone found out? It could be Dr. Boshaft, ULTRA's doctor. It could be the government that said EDTA is not completely approved for Western medical use. Do you think we got him in trouble?"

"Oh dear, I wonder," I said, shuddering at the thought. "I hope not. Let's not jump to conclusions. Everyone hits bumps in the road once in a while. It doesn't have to be all about us."

"Think about the timeline," Clint persisted. "In February, Dr. Tiens filled out that paperwork with the disability reason of 'heavy-metal toxicity.' He admitted treating me for work-related illnesses. He filled out that form. I read it. He said this was crossing the line. Maybe Dr. Boshaft has a connection here as well."

"Clint, we don't know for sure where the FDA stands on the use of EDTA, do we? We have been guessing all these months, based on the level of difficulty we've had getting any doctors to help. To us, it *seems* like the medical world is afraid to treat your conditions. Not one doctor has actually *said* that. Yes, a few did tell us to leave when we asked if they thought your problems were heavy-metal-related. But all we have is the emergency room doctor whispering that lifesaving piece of advice a year ago."

Then I stopped, realizing that I did know that the government was hiding facts about heavy-metal toxicity. I remembered an article concerning fracking and the Pennsylvania gag order that prohibited doctors from sharing information with patients exposed to toxic fracking solutions. The article claimed that when a doctor treated a patient who was multisymptomatic with issues that resembled poisoning, the doctor was not allowed tell the patient. Instead, he or she was to diagnose something commonly accepted and treat the patient accordingly, without revealing the underlying issue. The doctors were supposed to report this information to the government without the knowledge or consent of the patient.

This article on the internet from 2012 states:

Then-governor Tom Corbett's office said in 2013 it did not think the provision would bar doctors from freely speaking to their patients, but many health professionals interviewed by the media said the potential liability posed by the language of the law created too large a risk. The law is written in such a way, Jerry Silberman, a spokesperson for the Pennsylvania Association of Staff Nurses and Allied Professionals, told IB Times in 2012, that if a doctor thinks a patient suffers from symptoms brought about by fracking, the doctor isn't legally allowed to inform the patient of those suspicions. (http://fusion.net/story/353132/pennsylvania-supreme-court-gag-order-fracking)

There's HIPAA (the federal Health Insurance Portability and Accountability Act of 1996) again. How many times was I told that I could not talk to Clint's doctors or see any of his test results because of the HIPAA law? Then I found out that all of Clint's records were sent to a medical device company in Wisconsin that turned around and solicited Clint, suggesting he buy something that promised to stop his spastic bladder. This happened sometime around 2008. Returning to 2008 for a moment ...

2008

I answered my cell phone. It was Clint. "I just tried to use my credit card at the grocery store and was told my card's not active. I came home and called Capital One. Someone in Wisconsin has been using my card number. Capital One saw it and canceled the card. Another person's trying to use the card in India. How did this happen? I don't use my card on the internet. So how did someone get my credit card number?"

"How would I know?' I answered, only half listening.

A few days later, Clint got an invitation from a company located in Wisconsin to attend a seminar in Charleston regarding a medical miracle implant device that can stop bladder spasms. Apparently, Wisconsin (the same state where the credit card was being used) was where Clint's current urologist's office had sent his records.

Dr. Davidson, whose name appeared on the invitation, was not Clint's urologist but was a doctor in his urologist group. Certain of the source of the security breach with the credit card, I called the urologists' office.

Of course, the office denied sending away medical records, but I had the letter with Dr. Davidson's name on it. At the very least, there had been an inappropriate use of medical and financial information.

May 2012

"Mom, I am going to try to go work for a friend," Clint said. "We need the money, and I need to see if I can push through this. He'll be nice and understanding. I need to try. Maybe I need to get outside and sweat this stuff out." Clint was riding the section of the roller coaster that gave him time to breathe, the calm before the drop. The place where he could say, "I feel a little better!"

"Okay," I answered, wishing and hoping that this could work out for him.

Clint worked for a few weeks, but he only became sicker.

Dr. Tiens was no longer an option because no one answered the office phone any longer. When Clint looked through the windows of the office, it was empty.

My life was crumbling again. *Again?* I thought. *When did the crumbling stop so it could begin again?* I got up to go to work every morning and found myself crawling back into bed after my shower after getting dressed.

Garin, who had been encouraging me to take a vacation with him, suddenly changed his tune and started hounding me to see a physician myself. He was concerned, but his concern made me angry rather than comforted. Couldn't he see the urgency of the situation?

"Go! Take a vacation if you want, Garin! I'm needed here!" I told him in exasperation. "Go play golf or racquetball! Go surf or rodeo! If you cannot help, just stay out of the way!"

Clint was not looking good at all. The EDTA infusions had stopped, and Dr. Tiens's office looked half empty with records dumped on the floor looking like the FBI came through with a search warrant allowing them to create chaos with his patient's files.

Get up, get up! I told myself from under the covers. *You must stay strong. You have to fight through this. You keep telling Clint not to give up, yet here you are with your head stuck under the covers like a coward! You're being a baby. Do what you have to do. Get up!*

I crawled out of bed, feeling as if I could barely function. Perversely, I wished Garin was there to encourage me to see a doctor or to fly off on a vacation, so I could argue with him. But there was no way I could save Clint while Garin lived with us. Garin's views and mine were wildly disparate, and I needed to stay focused.

In truth, I was tumbling into depression. It had been two long, hard years since Clint had come home to die.

Why doesn't he just die, then, and get it over with? I thought uncharitably. But it was killing me to watch Clint suffer again. It was killing me not to be able to push him through to the other side. Some days it seemed like he was winning. That didn't last long, and he was soon falling apart again. I was perpetually exhausted; I was losing weight and looked bedraggled.

Damn it, I told myself. *Stop whining! You're not the one in pain. Get up and do something!*

Clint had stopped getting into the chamber. It caused him too much anxiety.

The MRI had come back good, showing the right hip had no necrosis and the left had a little. Dr. Khanna had said, "It may completely repair itself."

Clint's diet and supplements were important. We needed to get the lead out of the bones. We were trying, but we had hit a wall.

I went to see a friend, Suzanne, whom I hadn't seen for a long time. Actually, I could have said that about virtually all of my friends. I hadn't seen any of them for a very long time.

"How's Clint?" she asked when we were seated at her kitchen table, and our cups of green tea were steeping.

"Like in the past, Clint needs a change-up. These poisons keep outsmarting the detoxification plans. The secret to detoxification is change. Mix it up. Keep the neurons in the brain from getting tricked by the heavy metals by continually changing the process. I need a new process and a new doctor to tell me what I'm missing. Clint has been trying to figure it out by mixing his own supplements and DMSA and miso soup. I think we need someone who can give us a new idea."

"Have you ever heard of the Lumiere Metabolic Institute?" she asked.

My ears perked up. *What? A new idea? I thought all the new ideas were gone from the magic idea box. I thought I had used the last one. You mean there is one more left? Give it to me!*

Suzanne told me about her cousin's experience with Lumiere. "In six months, Sasha's symptoms were manageable. She was able to stop taking antidepressants and go back to school. She'll be graduating soon with a degree in chemistry, of all things. Her mother always suspected Benzene as the source of Sasha's neuropathy, and the girl only worked in that old factory over one summer."

Can they help Clint? I wondered as Suzanne continued talking and pointedly placed a cranberry muffin on my plate.

A sympathetic woman named Margie answered the phone when I called Lumiere the very next day. I told her the longest version of our story ever and how Clint was going backward. I explained my fear for his life and stressed that trouble seemed to be accelerating faster this time. My son had no reserves left.

"Mrs. Marshall …"

"Please call me Peggy."

"All right, Peggy. I can make an appointment for him," Margie said. "But we're six weeks out."

Unexpectedly, the warrior in me turned into a runaway deserter. I started to cry and stutter. "I—I, no, Clint can't wait that long," I pleaded. "Please. He's going down, and I don't know why. We had to stop the EDTA a couple of months ago for several reasons, and he's turning yellow again!"

"Don't cry," Margie consoled me. "Let me see if I can call someone. A patient scheduled for Friday may give up her appointment for you if I explain the situation. I'll call you back, Peggy."

When she called back an hour later, Margie had good news. "Would you like that Friday appointment?" she asked.

Smiling, perhaps maniacally, I added Margie to my Good People List. *Friday will be a new beginning,* I promised myself. But as I drove home that night, my own thoughts plagued me.

What happens if you get home and he's dead? What are you going to do then? Will you cry in grief? Will you cry in relief? What will you do? This despairing round of thoughts had asserted itself with increasing frequency until it seemed to haunt me all of the time. I felt like I was becoming a robot. I could hardly recognize myself in the mirror. Clint was scared and fully back in the business of dying.

What will tonight bring? I wondered as I pulled my car into the garage, the garage connected to my house of death.

I had a new doctor for Clint. We had another hope, another reason to go on. *Who's this doctor for, him or me? I wonder if I'm being totally selfish. Should I stop this search and help him die?* I wondered. But there he was, standing in the doorway, waiting for me to talk with him. *He's waiting for me to find the answers. I am his mom. Answers are what I do.*

"Hi, Clint," I said with as chipper a voice as I could muster. "I have some good news. Today I called the office of a doctor who specializes in metal toxicity. You have an appointment this Friday. I had to cry to get it. It wasn't pretty."

As I climbed the basement stairs, I thought, *I have cried more in the past four years than I have in my entire life previously.*

Clint looked at me, exhaustion overtaking his posture and features. "That's good, Mom. I will go if you think that is what I need to do."

Friday arrived in what seemed like the original six-week waiting period. Clint was back on his death-defying roller coaster, and I was back in my never-say-die warrior-from-hell existence. Off we rode into the early morning sun, hoping for a glorious get-out-of-death card.

Margie came out to meet us when we arrived. The richly appointed office was populated with anorexic-looking personnel. Margie was the exception. Close to my age, she seemed to emanate motherly instincts—and she seemed to understand me.

Lumiere Metabolic Institute treats medical conditions caused by poorly functioning digestive systems. I have come to learn that most medical conditions are caused by poorly functioning digestive systems. This means our food is toxic. Our environment is toxic. Our human bodies have become toxic. Our guts can no longer absorb the little nutrition available in the toxic foods that we ingest. Change the food choices. Fix the gut; fix the disease.

Lumiere treats obesity and other metabolic disorders. Heavy-metal toxicity becomes a metabolic disease. Thanks to Suzanne, once again Clint was pointed to a good place to be. As with others, this facility did not accept insurance. Every charge was out of pocket. I had come to understand that the medicine that worked for Clint was not covered under health insurance. I believe that is because it works. The doctors who do this type of healing probably don't want the government and health insurance companies to tell them what they can and cannot do to treat their patients. Therefore, it works.

Again, I base this on Clint's experiences with the medical world, and I believe I truly have the right to express my feelings and findings. After all, I was pretty much out of cash by this point. (And frankly, my retirement outlook is distant and sad.)

First, the doctor looked at my overstuffed three-ring binder that the Western doctors always refused to regard as medical fact. Reviewing this binder takes a lot of time, many minutes that would never be allowed in the Western medical world that takes insurance.

Then they used a controversial test called an electro dermal screening (EDS), for which I found mixed reviews on the internet.

Electric current flows through everyone's body, powering all vital functions. Meridians are channels connecting acupuncture points. The meridian system is based on diagnosis of these electrical pulses to reveal weaknesses in energy flow.

Clint was given a brass cylinder with wires that attached to a computer. As the doctor or his assistant placed a probe on his hands and feet, graph images depicting the strength of electric current pulses appeared on the monitor.

The EDS process involved the creation of an energy loop or electro-magnetic field. Bioactivity compounds or nutritional elements such as probiotics, magnesium, and calcium have their own electromagnetic field.

When supplements are placed on the testing plate while a person's own electromagnetic field is being tested, the positive or negative impact of each supplements can be measured.

On a brass place that was also connected to the computer, the doctor placed one after another tiny glass jar-like container, each holding a supplement Clint's body might need. As he placed a jar, his assistant would move the probe from meridian point to meridian point on Clint's hands or feet. The graph changed as jars were added and removed.

The doctor explained that when the brass plate was filled with what it would take to balance Clint's dying body, the graph lines on the screen would all be in balance with each other.

Serious voodoo here, I thought.

The doctor muttered dire comments regarding Clint's suppressed life currents and the magnitude of damage in his system. These were comments we had heard expressed in different words time and time again, including "We may be too late."

This doctor had no hospital privileges, and he was going to start Clint on a new wellness program that no Western medical world physician would respect. With death dogging Clint's heels, he was stepping further down a path marked "No Return."

The doctor determined a supplement list, including doses of the DMSA chelating element.

For a thousand dollars and a couple of hours of our time, we were out the door. Clint was to take 1,500 milligrams of DMSA over the weekend and do a twenty-four-hour urine collection for heavy-metals testing. Clint was given a large plastic jug to collect his urine while he took the DMSA. Strange; this was the same jug that the emergency room gave him in 2011.

Since DMSA is given as a chelating agent, this test is not accepted by the governmentally controlled medical world.

In a few days, the results came back, and were pretty much as expected. Clint was sick with heavy-metal poisoning and over body burden.

Clint decided to start another campaign toward healing, and Lumiere's program demonstrably helped in fewer than six weeks.

He followed every new rule while he continued to follow all the old rules. I still don't know how he did it. He was such a trooper through the entire discovery process. Clint did what Western doctors say they do—practice medicine.

Within six weeks, we were headed back to Lumiere for a progress report. Oh my God, the added help was amazing! My worries, though not gone, were immensely lessened.

The Lumiere staff confirmed with their testing device that Clint should be feeling better. His test results were amazing. His body was getting back in balance. The toxins were leaving his body and no longer digging in. Before arriving for the appointment, Clint already knew this was going to be the case. In just six weeks, he was feeling better.

August 2012

Clint and I celebrated the one-year anniversary of his decompression surgery. He still had bad days, but now he could work in the yard, cutting the grass. He did all of the grocery shopping and cooking, and he cleaned up the kitchen by himself.

I continued to work. Grams's trust supplied funding for the Lumiere visits. Thank goodness for that. I bought all the other special things Clint needed to stay well. Garin pitched in regularly, and my sisters and parents sent surprise money every once in a while. It always arrived just when we needed it the most.

Clint religiously worked out on his reformer two to four times a day.

Kit was amazing.

"She knows her stuff," Clint claimed after every visit.

He used his reformer. He sat and spun on his bike. He lifted weights and did pull-ups. Progress was slow and scary—but he was on his way back!

I cannot stress enough that heavy metals are smart. They take over the brain. A sick person has to have someone to help manage this process, someone like me to observe the daily changes and watch for the danger signs. The poisoned person can't see those. His or her brain is controlled by the alien metals.

The Haven Rehab Center was doing amazing things for Clint's hips. I paid for some, and Grams's trust money paid for some.

Kit was training, changing, and counseling Clint on the reformer.

Meg, bless her heart, ran every time Clint called. Some days she worked for an hour and a half straight, doing trigger-point release therapy, getting the toxins to release from one spot in his body. Then, two days later, Clint would return, and she'd do it again.

This is what it took to pull the toxins out through the skin. With Meg's amazing ability to know which muscles to twist and which soft tissue to press on, Clint usually felt better in fewer than three days. We felt like we had the perfect plan.

Somewhere between spring 2012 and July of that year, we made an amazing discovery. Most of Clint's groin pain was caused by swollen lymph nodes.

Years earlier, I had found an article about a race car driver who died of prostate cancer. I remembered that the article talked about metallic nanoparticles getting stuck in the lymph nodes, clogging them and causing swelling and extreme pain, the clogged lymph nodes eventually led to the man's death. Only then were the nanoparticles discovered. Remembering that article, I started searching the internet for information about lymph nodes and where they are located in the human body. Sure enough, most of Clint's extreme pain was around the places in his body that have the most lymph nodes.

Clint told Meg, and she began to do massage therapy to help remove the sludge from his lymph nodes. Along with that, he began to take more supplements that aid the lymph nodes in their work. The lymph nodes cleansing process only flows upward and toward the neck. Lymphatic system drainage is divided into two separate drainage areas. The right drainage center clears the right arm and chest. The left drainage center does the rest of the body. The tissues must be pinched and rolled toward the chest and neck when doing massages aimed at detoxifying the lymph nodes.

I wondered if Clint's left hip was worse than the right because the left lymph nodes had more areas to cleanse than the right. Again, I wished I was a doctor or that Clint had a doctor who would answer these questions. I wished we had a doctor who would just listen for five minutes.

Onward and upward, Clint was getting back on track. I couldn't have felt happier or more grateful.

October 2012

The day arrived. Clint had his answer explaining the mystery behind Dr. Tiens and Nurse Roberta when the following letter arrived in the mail:

October 1, 2012

Dear Patients and Friends:

For almost thirty years, quality patient care with a close doctor-patient relationship has been our goal.

Due to ethical differences with McClintock Memorial Hospital Administration we can no longer remain associated with Rosehill Medical Center. We will not compromise our patients' care, which is and always has been our top priority!

Therefore, with much sadness, we must close our medical center. Our last day of scheduled appointments will be October 25, 2012.

With hearts of gratitude, thank you for allowing us to serve you. It has been a blessing to us! You have touched our lives and become like "family." We want to assist you in locating a new family physician. Please visit the following websites to locate a board-certified family physician:

The Christian Medical and Dental Association—CMDA.org

The American Osteopathic Association—Osteopathic.org

Enclosed is a medical records release. Once you have located a new physician, please complete and FAX or mail it back to us. We will then be able to forward your records to your new physician. We will provide refills of your medications for thirty days to allow you time to locate a new family physician.

Please stay in touch with us. We will continue to expand our educational website, writing, research, advanced laboratory testing, and development of professional grade nutritional products. Nutritional health and preventive medical consultations will continue to be available by phone and e-mail. We will also produce educational videos and continue with speaking engagements.

We expect our phone number, FAX number, and e-mail addresses to remain the same for some time to come.

We continue to seek guidance from above. May God's grace continue to bless you.

Warmest Regards,

Marcel and Roberta Tiens

Another chapter in this story had come to an end. What do you think went wrong? One year after Dr. Tiens agreed to be Clint's doctor, he would be no one's doctor. It is now my understanding that private-practice doctors are being forced to join large hospital groups or be squeezed out. Because of the individualized treatment plan and time devoted to Clint and all of his patients, Dr. Tiens decided to leave the Western world of large money-making corporate America. His way of practicing medicine no longer fit the insurance companies' rules. I have a feeling that is why he closed his doors. What a very sad ending to the careers of a great, caring doctor and his devoted wife.

Fourteen

Healing Progress (2012–2014)

December 2012

"Thanks for dropping me off, Clint," I sang as he pulled his truck up to the curb at Yeager Airport. "I will be home in ten days."

I trusted that he wouldn't have to call me in pain. Because he hadn't worked since 2010, he wouldn't be calling to tell me that he had just gotten fired, as he had on the last Christmas I spent away from him.

Clint walked around to get my bag out of the truck. He looked remarkably better—not great and not pain-free but much improved.

"Bye, Mom," he said, giving me a big, happy grin that I remembered from so long ago. We had been through so much. Some days we fought and argued and bickered. Some days we were on the same bus of total agreement, heading straight to the land of painless days. Of course, we still tossed a coin to decide who got to drive the metaphorical bus. Some days were good. Some were not so good. I smiled back at him and gave him a big, healthy hug.

There were good days and bad days. I finally thought we might reach the point where we would get to good *years*, not just days.

January 2013

The changing weather threw Clint back into hip pain. Daily temperature fluctuations caused his swollen, heavy-metal-irritated tissues to throb. His body was healing, though, and it was not the worst he had ever been.

Just another bump in the road, I thought—and hoped.

We talked about moving down South where it was warm, and we wouldn't have to deal with such temperature fluctuations. But I didn't have any funds left. My work and our survival were here.

"Meg says she can fit me in tomorrow," Clint told me after calling her. "My hips are locking up again with this cold weather. I figure she can help reduce the swelling in my soft tissue and make some of this pain let up." He was using his reformer, trying to get his hips to let loose.

"Of course she can fit you in," I said with a confident smile. "Doesn't she always get you in the next day?"

My Good People list, I said to myself. *Let's think about this. There's Dr. Fritzmeyer, Meg, Kit, Kara, Tim, Haven Rehab, Lumiere, Dr. Tiens, and Nurse Roberta.* I thought again about the last two. *What a shame. I wonder what happened to Dr. Tiens and Nurse Roberta.*

As I went into my office to get back to work, I also remembered the bad people along the way. The people who didn't land on my happy list were more numerous than I cared to remember. I felt greatly fortunate to have found the good ones.

I wondered what had happened to Dr. Boshaft. I wondered if he spent any of his days worried that Clint hadn't died and might someday expose him. I smiled to myself. *I sure hope so.*

"Mom," Clint said, breaking into my thoughts. "Have I ever told you that this reformer is the best thing ever?"

"Just keep swimming," I sang with a laugh in my voice.

Sure, we still have bad days. But they don't last like they used to. We have learned what to do when the pain train comes roaring back to the station that we call home. Clint has gotten strong enough to bounce back. We have an A-1 team!

It's not a team that professes eternal pain and gloom. It's a group of caring, get-well professionals who know their specialties very well. They're not bottom-feeders like most of the Western-licensed physicians with whom we wasted so many years, hoping they would listen. Most of Clint's team members are not Western-licensed doctors.

Dr. Fritzmeyer is a chiropractic nutritionist who knows more than any MD. I am so glad that he chose healing the body versus passing out pills while killing it. When it comes to understanding the chemistry and biology of the human body, I will choose a Dr. Fritzmeyer over anyone else.

May 2013

"Mom, I want to try to go to work again," Clint said, as he had said every summer. When it got nice outside, he wanted to fully live. More than that, he wanted to be making a living. Yes, he had *really* good days, and I wanted to keep it that way.

He was still detoxifying. He had hip pain when the metals were on the move. He knew this. It had become predictable. It started out small. A not-so-great day might have been the beginning of the downward spiral. The heat could start it. Not eating on schedule and therefore not getting his supplements on time and in the correct order could cause it. Or maybe his body just needed to take a toxic dump. We didn't know. What I did know was that he was still sensitive to change. Change could set him up for some pain-filled days.

"Really, Clint?" I asked. "Are you sure you want to do this?"

"Yes! My friend's working for a guy who pours concrete patios. I can work when I want, and he promises to let me drink lots of water and take breaks so I can take my supplements. He says he understands and needs someone to help with the light work. I *need* to have my life back."

Clint went back to work for about three weeks. But the heat started breaking him down. He started hurting again. He quit the job and decided to take up fishing instead.

"Good idea," I said in total relief. He was disappointed; we both were. He had to try, and now we knew.

Clint no longer went to the Haven Rehab Center. His hips had enough strength and stability for him to work out on his own and with Kit.

"Mom, you should go with me sometime when I go fishing," he offered. "It's a group of lakes made from the gravel pits. There's sand and mud for me to slop through. The ground is uneven and rocky in some places. I have found a new place to rehab my hips. I'm finding out where I need strength. I need to work on that labrum that Dr. Savvin reattached. That hip wants to let go when I try to balance on uneven terrain. I have a fallen tree branch that I walk on like a balance beam.

"In the beginning, I couldn't make it across, toe to heel, without falling off. I made it today. I *made* it today! Do you *hear* me? It's too bad Lighthouse doesn't listen to me about rehabilitating hips. I could probably tell *them* what to do. More than that, I can tell them what *not* to do. Most of the *nots* are what they told me to do in the very beginning. I guess I'm glad Dr. Khanna refused to help me. I would *really* be disabled."

June 2013

Clint had been going to the Lumiere office to buy supplements but had not gone for a visit for a while. "Clint, maybe we need to see Dr. Lowell and see how you are doing. What do you think?"

Clint made the appointment and went without me. Since his days had been getting better, he didn't need me to tag along anymore.

But the appointment didn't go very well.

"How was Dr. Lowell?" I asked.

"Really off," Clint answered. I gave him a questioning look and he continued. "He didn't want to hear me. I tried to tell him what I've been doing. I tried to tell him what works and what does not work for me. He wrote everything down. Then he said what I am doing won't work. I asked him why—I am getting better! He didn't really answer that question. I wish you had come along. He was kind of mean and arrogant. I'm not going back. I don't need him. I just need his supplement source."

The rest of summer continued in a positive way. Clint rode the roller coaster: good days interspersed with painful days. But the roller coaster was no longer *monster huge*; it was a *monster light*, a kiddie version.

Clint continued to fish and to rehabilitate his hips at the lakes that connect with the Ohio River. He continued to work on the reformer two to three times a day.

October 2013

"Let's go," I said with a sigh. *Why are we doing this again?* We were going to visit our third disability attorney. *Here we go again,* I thought. I was driving to downtown Charleston with Clint sitting next to me. We were doing the same thing we had done over and over again, expecting different results. *This is actually the definition of insanity. How stupid are we? Dr. Khanna still won't help. No one understands what four hip surgeries in eleven months will do to a person. No one understands Clint's pain. Worst of all, our government refuses to recognize heavy-metal poisoning as a disabling disease.*

The disability attorney wanted Clint to change his claim from hips to mental issues or back pain. Sadly, we had enough medical history to support either one.

"Back or mental issues," the disability attorney told us. "You can get disability with one of those. If you stick with this hip thing, you simply will not win. The government never argues over crazy because they cannot disprove crazy. Be crazy, and get your money."

Clint stood tough (maybe stupidly tough but tough). "I am working *very* hard to beat this. Let's say I do claim to be crazy and then try to get a job. My potential employer asks me if I'm crazy to want to come back to work as a piper. What will I say if I go after the crazy card to get disability? If I say no, then I guess I lie. If I say yes, then I guess I will have to stay on disability forever and continue to be crazy. Either way, *this* is crazy. I *am* hurt. I got hurt on the job. There has to be justice in this world."

There does not! I thought. *Or if there is, I haven't seen it.*

Clint was given eighteen months of disability income. There's a disability qualifying rule that states, "Any person who stays on crutches consistently without a break qualifies for disability for that twelve-month period, no more, no less, through the rehabilitation period." Since Clint was on crutches from August 31, 2010, through September 2011, he was granted the twelve months plus six months for rehabilitation.

Several times, Dr. Khanna was served a subpoena to show up in court. He never did. He didn't have to. I don't know why they even wasted the time on the subpoenas.

We had to wait for that first check until December 31. The disability attorney received a large part of the settlement—and I added another bottom-feeder to my Black Hats list.

November 2013

Clint was still detoxifying. In 2010, Clint had needed drastic, immediate, lifesaving measures. It was dangerous, and Dr. Fritzmeyer was cautious. But Clint had been dying. Throwing caution to the wind, we had made a potentially deadly decision. Clint was lucky. The way we chose worked.

In November 2013, Clint went back to Dr. Fritzmeyer to finish up this long road back to health.

Heavy-metal disease finally has a name: TILT, or toxicant-induced loss of tolerance. I am immeasurably glad that someone has taken the time to study and give respect to the people who severely suffer from this often-undiagnosed illness.

That's the beginning of the silver lining.

At first, I wanted to write this book to reach all the sick construction workers from the ULTRA renovation. Then I wanted to write this book for all the pipe fitters and welders who are being exposed to heavy metals every day on job sites across America. Then I wanted to write this book because I thought someone took down my dear Dr. Tiens and Nurse Roberta. Then I wanted to write this book because I was angry with the Western doctors. Then I wanted to write this book because no matter how hard I tried to explain what happened in this house and how Clint saved his own life, no one gets it. As I finish writing this book, maybe I am doing so to help everyone. TILT is not just caused by work exposures. I am discovering that it has many different causes. I am trying to tell people to take charge of their medical treatments, to listen to their bodies. If your doctor doesn't listen to you, and he or she prescribes drugs without looking for ways to first help your body heal itself, *run* away. I truly believe that if a person takes pharmaceutical drugs, the disease is given a free ride to run amok and create other disease. We all know the game. More drugs, more disease. Trust me; in most cases your body can fix itself. Find a doctor who can discover the root cause, and give yourself the time that it takes to rebalance itself. Find a health coach who can help you monitor your progress. As with Clint, an ill person cannot be the judge of positive or negative changes. Keep a diary of how you feel every day. Good or bad, it is so important to record what is happening. What did you eat? How much water did you drink? Were you able to sleep? Keep a daily record of your pain level. It is especially important to keep track of your mental health. What did your brain tell you today? Were you in a positive mood, or was your day filled with fear? Your state of mind controls your ability to heal. That is why you need a coach.

Somewhere in all of this, many people have reached out to me, asking for help regarding heavy-metal poisoning and autoimmune disease. I know of one person specifically who returned to 95 percent complete wellness. The last time I talked with him, he called me *his* angel. That is another reason for this book.

I believe the biggest reason for this book, though, is to encourage parents of children who are diagnosed with learning disabilities to not just accept what their doctors say. Food and lifestyle choices can make a difference. Drugs kill the liver, weaken the immune system, and unbalance the brain. I don't want this to happen to their children.

Now that most of the story is finished, let me go back to the beginning.

Remember when I first said that Clint was born with five learning disabilities? Remember when I said that Clint could not auditorily process words? He couldn't spell. He could hardly read, and he couldn't break words into syllables. He couldn't hear letter sounds or groups of letters that make up words. Clint had to have perfect silence when he watched TV, or he could not understand the words.

As hard as he tried, he could not learn to read above a fifth-grade level. As hard as he tried, he couldn't learn algebra or geometry. Math was not a big deal, as most things formulated in his head. He was able to travel all over the United States to get to jobs because of his incredible coping skills and—now identified—high IQ. He could hang pipe without the use of a calculator or knowing formulas. The drop lengths and pipe angles formed in his head as he looked at the space.

Get ready; *this* is the interesting part of the story. As Clint continued through his detoxification process, he started to hear word sounds. He started to hear syllables in words. He started to hear consonants and vowels. He was quite excited when this started happening. It's like having a baby who is learning to walk. He never knew that the constant *shhhhhh* in his head was not normal until the day it disappeared. As the *shhhhhh* disappeared, his ability to spell and read began to take its place.

Clint went to Kentucky to visit a work buddy in April 2014. When he returned home, he came running into my office, screaming, "I can *spell Kentucky.* I can *hear KEN-TUCK-EEE.*" He was so excited; I thought he was going to pee his pants. He must have spelled Kentucky for ten minutes straight, standing right behind me, yelling in my ear.

A few days later, when I came home, he met me at the door with a huge grin on his face. "Listen to this, Mom, I can hear and spell *mac-a-roni.*" For the following fifteen minutes, he repeated over and over again how to spell *Kentucky* and then *macaroni.*

Clint had never been able to hear letter sounds. He carried a notebook with him just in case he had to spell the days of the week or months of the year. Filling out job applications at the beginning of his career was a white-knuckle experience. After a few times, he was able to memorize the forms in general, and he was okay.

Two weeks ago, he learned the word *ability. A-bil-i-ty.* Having seemed to have turned into a walking spelling bee contestant, he was spelling every word he could that had *ability* in it. That is such an ironic word for him to choose if you think about what he was able to do. My LD, self-esteem-destroyed son was gaining the *ability* to read. CAMC Women and Children's Hospital's word on this had been *never*.

For thirty-eight years, Clint was disabled. Over the past twelve months, he had become an entirely new person. He was reborn! He smiled and carried on conversations with family members for whom he never would've had a word in the past. His short attention span and quick-to-anger personality had vanished.

He was always hiding because of his inability to understand words. Social gatherings had been extremely painful for him. When he was in seventh grade, he described his life like this: "There's a monster out there. This monster can ruin my life by exposing my stupidity. I know he's behind every single door I pass. I'll never escape him." It broke my heart. He had always tried so hard to learn.

Through the doors of near death, the person I had always known was in there exploded from his broken-down, hollowed-out body.

I've previously stated the following, but it bears repeating:

According to science, we can now reverse the damage that may have been caused by environmental toxins. Since the brain has the capacity to rewire itself and form new neural pathways, you can improve the brain functioning by treating your brain in a healthier manner. For example, the mere effect of food alone on the brain is so powerful that the foods you eat can affect your moods.

Since November 2013, Clint has attended every family holiday event. He went to more family events in one year than he previously had attended in his entire life. My family still cannot believe what they see.

Sad note: I try hard to convince parent, who are doing the battles of life with their neurologically challenged children that there is another road to travel, a different bus to get on. I explain some simple changes they can make in daily choices pertaining to food and supplements. They all think my story is interesting but that it cannot possibly be as bad as what they are living today. They think their special situations are much different from mine, that what I say will never work for them. What do they fear?

Then again, in June 2014, the FDA took away the only supplement that breaks through the brain barrier to remove neurotoxins. I will say it again; I will scream it if I have to. The government poisons us while they take away the only thing Clint had to get well!

Was Clint born poisoned from the well water that collected from the DDT-sprayed cornfield where we lived? Our shallow well drained into the neighbor's lake that they used to water their crops. Our well would run dry, and we would have the local water truck dump water into the well. The water was muddy and most likely toxic. Did I poison my child? As I already stated, we moved when Clint was eighteen months old. I have to wonder what happened to that piece of land before we moved in.

I also wonder how toxic the vegetables were that the next-door neighbor grew and sold to the local market. Ugh. How far do environmental toxins reach? We will never know.

Clint still has not qualified for disability. He cannot work, though he has tried several times. Every time, he slides backward.

Diet, rest, and physical therapy on a rigorous schedule generally obviate serious pain.

He never has taken pain meds. He refuses, even on his worst days.

He looks fabulous, so no one guesses he was ever sick a day in his life. After four invasive back-to-back hip surgeries and a back surgery in the summer of 2015, he walks without a limp or any sign of body destruction.

In 2013, Clint began West Virginia's program that helps disabled people find work. After he was tested for physical challenges and disabilities and then tested for skill-level abilities, the program administrators decided that he only qualified to be a parking garage attendant. Perhaps he could work at a uniform company doing laundry.

I researched the named uniform company that they suggested and found out that the government pays that company to hire people like

Clint. Other than those types of opportunities, the government workforce employees had nothing to offer.

Again, follow the money.

Clint cannot sit for longer than fifteen minutes at a time, cannot stand for longer than fifteen minutes at a time. He cannot stoop or bend or pick up more than ten pounds.

Yet they sent him on interviews that required heavy lifting and exposure to chemicals. He cannot work in a parking garage, as the job requires eight hours of sitting on an uncomfortable chair while being exposed to car exhaust fumes.

He cannot do laundry, which requires much stooping, bending, and twisting.

Furthermore, most of the potential employers were afraid to hire him. Who in their right mind would accept the liability of that potential worker's comp claim?

Clint asked the testing center if they thought he could use his pipe-fitting experience to be trained to draw the pipe layout before it goes into the field to be installed. They said no. They said he was not smart enough. His skill level and learning disabilities would not allow him to learn to be a detailer. But that was before he could spell and hear *ability*. This waste-of-time process took eighteen months—another government agency that serves no purpose.

In August 2015, Clint began taking a class at the community college. He asked permission to audit the class, just to learn the skill, not get a grade. He wanted to see if, once again, the professional, educated decision makers could be proven wrong.

Clint is a natural for AutoCAD, a design and drafting software application. He struggles. He doesn't have the book-taught math skills. He had never turned on a computer before August 2015. He never played computer games as those require reading abilities. What Clint has is true grit, the kind that the "last American cowboy" needs to have in order to survive.

The first class ended on his birthday, December 12, 2015, when Clint turned forty years old. He became sick when he was twenty-seven.

Clint now goes to college. He decided that the professional, educated decision makers were all wrong again—surprise, surprise! Only time will tell.

His second class is getting more difficult. Clint has great coping and workaround skills. He prints out the drawing and gets out his pipe-fitting measuring tools and pretends that he is going to hang the pipe. He figures out what is wrong and then fixes it in the computer program. In his first class, he earned a B—the first B in his life. All he ever got in fourteen years of school were Ds and Fs, which represent Dummy and Failure in a learning-disabled world.

In January 2016, he signed up for another class, saying, "I really like to learn." Who would have ever thought Clint's mom would hear those words? He plans on taking another when this one ends. He says if he doesn't learn this class well enough, he will take it again. Then he will take another.

It seems strange to me that our government will give handouts to those who don't want to try to change. Clint keeps asking just for temporary life enhancements while he struggles to get well and improve his future. He is denied, yet he undeniably has done virtually the impossible. He chose life without pain meds. He chose to fight for his life.

When Drs. Tiens and Fritzmeyer said that Clint most likely was over body burdened by the world he lived in, I made a search on my PC. I asked that any articles that contained *heavy metal, arsenic, over body burden,* and *toxins* be sent as an alert on my PC.

Articles began to flow in. Many people with Clint's symptoms were asking for answers to their supposedly psychosomatic chronic pain. I answered many of their questions, and we spent months talking on the phone and emailing each other. All—and I mean all—had the same story as Clint. Most had no money left. Believing the medical doctors, their families had given up on them. Moms and dads just walked away, refusing to listen and unable to understand. Many of these suffering individuals had no one to help them. They have environmental poisoning from all kinds of exposures. Some began right after they graduated from college when they had to get numerous vaccinations to accept jobs in the medical field. Some symptoms began after they were given the vaccine for Lyme disease. Some began with endometriosis and pelvic-floor dysfunction after having a difficult time during pregnancy and childbirth. One gentleman's hair test result came back with extreme platinum toxicity results. He had worn platinum glasses since he was in grade school.

It is sad that I know of only one person who has recovered. This person had lots of support. He was able to keep working while he listened to my suggestions and decided which ideas best fit his needs. He lived close enough to me that he was able to travel to see Clint's doctors. His family coached him and helped him identify the small progress that he made in each step of his wellness path.

I figure most of the people who called me are still suffering or have died, while the Western world of medicine blames their symptoms on something they did. Perhaps they died because the government is part of a huge cover-up, as they are in too tight with big business and money makers. Their pockets are lined with the money made at the expense of our children.

During the Christmas weeks in 2014, my father became very sick with bronchitis. He never recovered and declined rapidly. He died in April 2015. I felt so horrible. For the past seven years I had been so busy that I didn't get to spend much time with him. Another bundle of guilt and regret was added onto my back. Life just slips away.

Everyone was at my dad's funeral—all my family and friends. Out of the corner of my eye I saw someone who looked familiar. As hard as I tried, I could not recognize that person. One of my sisters asked me if it was Garin who had just come in. My heart dropped to my feet. I had seen Garin over Christmas, and he looked fine. Not so by April. His skin was gray, and he held his side as he shuffled his feet.

"Garin, what is wrong. You must be sick. You must have been sick for a while. Why didn't you call me?"

Garin forced his big-brother smile and replied, "You are so busy. I know what it's like to lose a parent. It would not have been fair to add another patient and worry to your list. I had to come and show everyone that I care and love them. I need them to know how sorry I am about their loss."

Garin sat down in a chair a few rows behind my family in the chapel. Clint and I sat beside him for the ceremony. My family totally understood and didn't say a word about our not sitting with them in the first row, where we were assigned. Garin left immediately after the dedication. Stooped and wobbling, he exited through the side door.

My war-torn warrior body was mentally suiting up. I had lots to do and apparently very little time. *I am so exhausted. Where am I going to find the power to accept another mission?* I asked myself. I said another prayer and told myself, *You can do it!*

For the moment, I had to get back into the present. Guests had to be consoled. The sisters needed to be a team. Garin would have to wait a day.

Clint was really grieving. "Mom, I am so angry. Life is so unfair. I can finally go to family functions and fit in. Grandpa and I were getting to know each other. We have so much in common. He loved to fish. I loved listening to his fish stories. He gave me all of his fishing stuff last summer. I promised to come and take him fishing this year, and now he is gone. I will never be able to go fishing with my grandpa. I brought one of his fishing poles today. I want Grandpa to take this fishing pole with him to heaven. That way when I fish, I can imagine Grandpa fishing next to me, holding this fishing pole. Do you think Grandma will let me do this?"

Tears filled my eyes. I swore that this warrior would not cry in front of my family and friends. I kept blinking and blinking. "Oh, Clint" was all I could say.

Clint went outside to get the fishing pole. I went to say goodbye to my dad. Clint came in and asked Grandma if he could put the fishing pole in with Grandpa. There was not a dry eye in the house.

Garin spent weeks in the hospital with the diagnosis of pancreatitis. "Please, Garin, allow me to manage your care. Let me talk with the doctors. What tests are they running? What are the doctors saying? You are sick. You need someone to be your advocate."

"Now, Peggy, let's let the docs do their job. They are taking care of me. They have a plan, and everything is going to be fine." Since Garin and I were not married, I was not automatically allowed to become his caretaker.

Good ole Garin. He always thinks people are his best friends and that everyone does his or her job without being pushed to perform. I had to say okay and remain his friend, knowing that his point of view was not my reality.

Garin was in and out of the hospital several times. Most of the time, he just lay in bed with an IV in his arm. He was not allowed to eat any food. Pancreatitis continued to be the diagnosis, with no other tests taken to look for a different cause. He just lay there, patiently waiting for something to change. Since doctors don't treat their patients in hospitals anymore, Garin's care was left in the hands of hospitalists. They did nothing except visit him every morning and record his vitals. They charged him for a doctor visit but did absolutely nothing to deserve their fee.

In June, I insisted that Garin move in with me. He protested, but he came. He was losing weight and couldn't eat anything. Finally, his gastrointestinal doctor agreed to run a few tests and acted so surprised when he announced that Garin had pancreatic cancer. Garin had been deathly sick for six months before the doctor ran tests for cancer. How does this happen?

This is my point of view, so maybe I'm wrong. In October 2014, Garin's health insurance premium rose to over seven hundred dollars a month. He'd never used his Cadillac insurance plan into which he had paid since 1995. He was never sick. He semiretired in spring of 2014 and, because of financial reasons, gave up his Anthem plan. He purchased an Obama "affordable" bronze health insurance plan. I say affordable sarcastically.

Once cancer was diagnosed, I began to look for the best cancer treatment center I could find. Garin's insurance was not accepted at most hospitals. The best-rated oncology group accepted his health insurance plan, but the hospital testing lab where they practiced would not. This makes no sense, as the oncologist did not accept lab or diagnostic test results from outside labs. How can a sick person choose an oncology group that is covered by insurance and pay out of pocket for lab and diagnostic services? Therefore, that practice was not a possibility. I believe this is a well-thought-out plan by the oncology group so they don't have to accept Obama health insurance. Garin was left with no choices. There was no special cancer care for Garin. The only oncologist that accepted Garin's insurance went through the process of attempting to appear to care. She did not.

Garin's sisters and I took turns taking him to his chemotherapy treatments. He kept losing weight. He became weaker and weaker. I kept asking his oncologist to get involved, to think outside the box. Can we please try some functional treatments to enhance their treatments? I argued with them with no positive results. They told us that if Garin chose alternative medicine it would interfere with his chemo. Garin would get so angry with me. He asked me to stop demanding answers. I decided to give up. If Garin wasn't in the fight, then neither was I. Sadly, there was nothing I could do. I cooked special food and tried to make him comfortable.

Garin died on October 1, 2015. Sadness filled this house. I was so guilty. I am sure I could have done something.

Fifteen

Stem Cell Therapy (2015-2017)

Previously I mentioned that on November 4, 2005, Clint received a prescription for Flexeril (a muscle relaxant). His back was showing "minimal degenerative changes in the lower spine."

In early 2015, Clint began getting cramping pain in his calf. The pain spread down into his ankle and foot. After several weeks of trying to figure out what was wrong, it was discovered that it originated in his spine. In July 2015, Clint underwent a discectomy procedure. This turned out to be a wrong turn down the bumpy road of surgery. He spent the rest of 2015 rehabbing his back.

In early 2016, Clint's back pain came back. The bulging disc that was "repaired" in July 2015 continued to be his battle—such disappointment and pain returning after such a short period of feeling better. Once again, we were off to doctors and surgeons who practiced Western medicine.

The prognosis was not good. "Clint's lower back needs to be fused" was the opinion of the surgeon who already had his chance in 2015. All I could see was a reflection of dollar bills when I looked into his eyes. "It will be a simple fix," he said. "No problem. We will fuse the disc and reinforce it with titanium screws."

You'd better believe I asked, "What happens if a person is sensitive to titanium?"

The surgeon didn't even ask me why that would matter. He was so arrogant that he just knew that titanium doesn't hurt anyone. He was ready to set up the surgical procedure as soon as he could clear his schedule. *Cha-ching!* Recurring income for the next ten years. Until death of his patient do they part. Clint is the perfect patient; he doesn't have an affordable Obama insurance plan, and Grandma pays his $650 monthly premium from his health trust fund.

Thanks, Gram.

In June 2016, I began making bone-broth soup from organic free-range chicken bones. Through my search for feeding a body back to health, I discovered articles about this magic potion. Bone broth is supposed to increase stem cells, reduce inflammation, and boost the immune system, among many other things. Clint began drinking about two cups of this broth a day.

By July, Clint was not able to walk more than twenty-five feet without extreme pain. He was lying on the floor on ice and heat for most of his days. The discogram showed the L4–L5 spinal disc was 50 percent reduced in height. This in itself is not a problem, but the disc was gray in color and extremely weak. It had a bulge, stenosis, and bone spurs directly touching the nerves.

Clint and I spent hours debating what we knew would be a horrible medical disaster. He had two other discs that were 85 percent of their original height. If we fused the worst disc, it was inevitable we would have to fuse the others. This was a no-win situation.

The surgeon's plan didn't happen. In the past year, we'd heard more stories about professional athletes repairing their backs, shoulders, and knees with stem cell therapies. Because of these stories, I began researching PRP and adipose fat stem cell therapy. I spent hours on the internet, reading though pages and pages of medical information. Most articles I could not understand. The ones I could led me where I needed to go next. I repeated what I had done in 2010, when I was looking for answers to Clint's pain. This new search took me about two weeks. Next, I had to find a stem cell clinic. This took a lot of time and hard work. I made appointments with a few doctors close to home. They didn't meet my expectations. I didn't stop. I knew stem cells were the answer. I found a pain-management doctor who was doing a stem cell research project twenty minutes from our house. This doctor completed all the required tests, but Clint didn't qualify for the research study. He didn't have enough increased pain when the discogram was done. Clint has a huge pain threshold. He proved this when he kept working with torn labrums in 2010. Again, things happen for a reason. Clint wasn't sold on the idea of signing on for a two-year research commitment and a possible placebo. We agreed to allow this doctor to treat his disc with PRP and forget the stem cells.

While Clint waited for the doctor to fit him into his schedule, I continued to search for a stem cell center. In my heart, I knew that was the answer. Perseverance paid off again. I found a stem cell facility ninety minutes from our house. I called the office and talked with the office person. Within minutes, I knew this was the doctor I had been looking for. I sent all of Clint's records. I knew Clint was in too much pain for a three-hour round-trip journey to meet and greet a doctor. I talked for about thirty minutes with the doctor's surgical nurse. She agreed that a pre-stem cell appointment didn't make sense. She made two appointments for Clint in one day. First, Clint would meet with the doctor, and they would discuss the procedure. He would examine Clint at ten thirty in the morning. At that appointment, he would decide whether Clint was a suitable candidate for stem cell therapy. If he felt Clint would benefit from the process; lipo-aspiration to pull stem cells from him would begin at one o'clock that afternoon. After the lipo-aspiration, blood would be drawn from Clint's arm. The blood would be spun and separated. PRP stands for platelet rich plasma. PRP is the body's repairing soldiers. They are the first responders when the body is injured. I understand they cause inflammation and make the blood clot so we don't bleed to death. They make repair ladders to which stem cells attach. The stem cells attach, grow, and multiple while repairing the damaged area.

In order to obtain the stem cells, fat must be taken from the abdomen by a needle and syringe aspiration. Fluid with numbing medication can be injected before the fat is removed with a syringe. The fat is dissolved, and the stem cells are obtained and then mixed with the patient's PRP, which is obtained from the blood. After the stem cells have been processed and mixed, they are injected into the affected disc in the same manner as any other joint injection.

Clint decided it was best to try the stem cell therapy. On September 14, Clint and I drove the ninety minutes to repair the major disease in his L4–L5 disc.

I found myself, once again, sitting in a waiting room, trying to breathe and stay calm.

I knew Clint was being put though extreme pain. The stem cells need to be pure. The doctor offered Clint a mild pain medication. Clint said, "No. This has to work. I don't want any possibility of harming my stem cells." Clint had liposuction with no pain meds.

The poor doctor worked for more than an hour and finally had to settle for three-fourths of the required fat. Not only did he try in Clint's abdomen, he also suctioned from his waist down into his butt cheeks. No fat could be found. We needed to treat all three discs, but Clint hardly had enough fat to repair just one disc. Much to his surprise, he told me that he obtained more stem cells from that small sample then he sees from his other patients. I just grinned. I knew it was the bone-broth soup and the other supplements that his functional doctor prescribed. I didn't share my secret to success because now all I cared about was Clint growing fat as fast as he could.

The precious stem cells were injected into the L4–L5 disc. "The other discs will have to wait," the doctor said with a deep, sad sigh.

As I searched on the internet for stem cell therapy and spinal disc rehabilitation, there was more negative information than positive. To that I say, when your achy back is up against the wall, and the surgical choices will soon leave you with no choices, what do you have to lose? Get on the *body-heal-thyself bus*, and go for it.

By November, Clint was walking two miles at a time, twice a day. Each day was filled with a fear of the unknown. Each week seemed to be a positive step forward, with days in between that made us question our decision. We continued to start each day with a positive attitude.

At the end of January 2017, Clint had another lipo-aspiration and stem cell transplant appointment. The doctor again hoped to collect enough fat cells to treat all three discs. Once again, he could not harvest enough fat from Clint. Clint tried to grow fat. It just doesn't happen that easily.

"Clint," the doctor said, "you have a problem."

"Just add it to my list," Clint said, "Now what?"

"I suggest that you allow me to send the fat that I was lucky enough to harvest to a lab that can grow them. You will need four more stem cell injections, but I cannot get enough cells to do that. This lab doesn't enhance cells with growth hormones, which could cause autoimmune disease."

Clint's face fell. We both knew that this was going to be expensive. He looked at me. What else could I say? It was working, so we had to keep going. We were back on the roller coaster, falling to the bottom of the huge hill. Although my mind was spinning I smiled. "Clint, you know we are in this to win. You are not a quitter. You do the healing, and I cover the cost, right?"

"Here's what I suggest," the doctor said as he cautiously drew in a nervous breath. "Let me feed your discs with PRP today. Your fresh blood platelets will enrich the discs to accept the stem cells in six weeks."

We completely trusted our doctor, so the blood was drawn, and his platelets were injected into three of his discs. The small amount of fat containing Clint's precious stem cells was sent to the growth lab. Again, there is no guarantee that his cells would grow. All we have is faith. We will run with that and keep on going.

I also have to recognize what damage this battle has done to me. By the end of 2015, I too was having health issues. I made an appointment with my doctor. I should have known better. She diagnosed high blood pressure. Glucose levels labeled me as prediabetic. I tried to explain that my dad had died in April, and Garin had died in October. I tried to tell her I thought it was not as simple as high blood pressure. I tried to tell her that I was suffering from adrenal exhaustion and inflammation. She refused to listen. She prescribed a medication that, once started, I would be taking for the rest of my life. I was headed down the self-poisoning-with-prescription-drugs path of no return. Soon, I would be treating more body failure with more self-poisoning prescription drugs.

I tried to believe my doctor, but something seemed to be wrong with her simple diagnosis. I never stopped feeling bad. After fifteen months of taking Lisinopril, I emailed Clint's functional doctor on a Friday night. He returned my email the next day—Saturday. We talked on Monday, and he ordered three organic tests. "I do not recommend you stop taking your Lisinopril. Your doctor feels that you need this. According to the test results, however, you don't have high blood pressure. Your hormone levels are out of balance. Your liver is not functioning as it should. The past ten years have exhausted your immune system. Your extreme fight-or-flight response has caused dangerous inflammation. This is causing internal pressure and anxiety." He sent me five supplements that he felt would balance my system and help relax my vascular system. I purchased a blood pressure cuff.

"You need to balance your hormones with diet adjustments. While you balance your hormones, the anxiety and brain fog that you are experiencing must be controlled with protein. Snack all day long on high-protein food." Surprise, surprise the anxiety stopped. I was able to sleep again. I began to feel better.

Present Day

Clint's back is steadily improving. It truly is an amazing process to watch. He is able to do a few push-up and can hold a plank position for about one minute. He is spinning on his bike for a few minutes each day. He is stretching on his reformer. He is always rehabbing. He never stops. He's a determined human machine.

Next Tuesday the stem cells will be ready. Everything is working as planned. Two weeks ago, I placed the stem cell order. Once again, I feel confident that Clint and I made the right decision. He is mostly out of pain. No titanium screws or plates in his back. His body is healing itself. Clint has a stem cell bank of his own to use whenever his body needs to be regenerated.

We continue to see recovery, and if the stem cells fail, we will find another miracle. I always say, "Decisions today control available choices in the future, so decide carefully."

Afterword

To look at Clint today, you can't tell what he has been through. Tall and handsome, he looks strong, confident, and healthy. If you didn't know his story, you'd never guess he's had so many surgeries that we've lost count. He stands tall and walks without any sign of previous trauma.

Clint and I now have indisputable proof that neurological issues can be chemically induced. I hope others will be able to use our journey to build recovery for themselves. I look forward to the day when there is a widely accepted protocol to liberate and elevate other people who suffer with TILT.

Warning: Self-prescribing supplements is very dangerous. Everyone is different. Extensive testing has to be done in order to determine what is out of balance and causing your symptoms. It is a science that requires highly trained professionals to order the tests, read them, and determine what will heal you. Taking the wrong combination of supplements can make you sicker.

All supplements are not equal. Research the manufacturer before you buy. Ask where the supplements are made. Are they pure? Some may have toxins and cause more harm than good. Some may have fillers. In order for a body to absorb and use the nutrition in a supplement, it has to come from food. The vegetables and minerals have to be processed without chemicals or high heat. More pharmaceutical companies are joining the supplemental sales club. They are secretly buying established supplement manufactures. They keep the original ingredients and branding while they maintain the market share. Over a short period of time, they change the ingredients, and you don't even know. Soon your supplements are not what they appear to be. They steal shelf space at natural food stores and force the business owner to replace the preferred brands with theirs. Trust me; I am not making this up. Again, follow the money.

The best advice is to take the supplements that your functional doctor advises and buy those supplements through your doctor. Internet sites are selling contraband. They are copying a supplement bottle label and selling supplements that are not supplements at all.

The best suggestion I can offer before you begin taking any supplemental program is this: Buy a book written by Mary Frost, *Going Back to the Basics of Human Health*. I cannot begin to share her wealth of information. When I first saw the book, I was suspect, as she is so committed to Standard Process brand supplements. She supports all of her feelings, however, with provable information. We didn't use Standard Process to detox Clint. We did use high-quality supplements made by reputable manufacturers.

I am finding trust again in Clint's future. I am once again allowing myself to have hope.

I relax every once in a while and almost forget the past ten years.

I find myself mentally removed from my body, sitting on the top of a mountain, high up on a ledge, overlooking a vast canyon. The eagles are soaring overhead, and I am calm. The ending to my book will not be an easy write, as my story is not really ended. Life just keeps on going with new challenges every day. My son is getting better physically, yes, but his mental fear will never leave him. Every little twinge in his body sends him down memory lane. Is this natural? Is this another detoxification symptom? Is this a disease finally coming to fruition? After all, every doctor told him he would die any minute or very soon from cancer, liver disease, or a heart attack. It's like a ticking time bomb as his heart continues to beat, pushing blood throughout his war-torn body.

We are still mending his back and hips, and the bills never stop. Insurance still refuses to pay for all of the medical choices we make. We have proven they work. Someday stem cells will be paid for by insurance. Until then, Clint is the money-pit guinea pig, testing the possibilities of body regeneration through alternative medicine.

Clint will never give up. He is the last American cowboy.

Is It Metal Poisoning? Your First Steps

Something just doesn't feel right. Your head feels like it's floating. You feel disconnected from life and friends. You don't breathe in as deeply as you have in the past. Your chest is tight. The things that you like to do no longer motivate you to participate in life. You have unexplained aches and pains. You have trouble sleeping.

A fifteen-minute appointment with your doctor results in a quick assessment. Your doctor orders diagnostic tests so she can confirm her diagnosis. She prescribes a couple of drugs and instructs you how to take them. "Don't miss a dose. Don't stop taking them until I say. Doctor's orders," she says. Your doctor refuses to listen to you. The fifteen-minute appointment doesn't allow for unnecessary conversations. Entering your symptoms into the laptop takes precedence over that silly stuff. You have to talk about your symptoms in order to obtain the required insurance code for treatment. That's all that really matters.

Your feeling of well-being doesn't return. You blame yourself, and you try harder to follow your doctor's explicit directions. You still don't feel any better. You try to call the doctor for a quick discussion, and you are told you have to come in for another fifteen-minute visit that will certainly begin thirty to forty-five minutes after the appointment time. By the time you get in to see the doctor, your nerves are shot, and your brain is waffling. She takes your blood pressure. "Oh my, no wonder you are not feeling well. You have high blood pressure," she says. She prescribes anxiety medication to help with your newly diagnosed depression.

If you are not getting the answers that make sense, and what they are selling you isn't worth buying, then it is time to try a different road to wellness.

It's time to take charge of your health. Doctors and medical facilities used to be about the art of practicing medicine. Now it's all about the art of making money and staying within the guidelines of insurance reimbursements.

Here is what I've discovered through my experience of looking for health answers that make sense:

If you have been unwell for a while and nothing seems to work to feel better, talk to your friends. Begin a health diary.

Write down what you remember about the first day of the symptom.

If you have not done so yet, make a fifteen-minute appointment with your doctor, and have the necessary tests done.

Keep a diary about everything, even if it seems insignificant.

Follow up with a functional doctor. Finding a functional doctor is not easy. I searched on the internet and called many offices. Most of the time, you can get a feeling if they will fit your personality by the way they respond to your questions.

If possible, visit the office. If the office staff looks like a Barbie doll convention, it's probably not a good fit for getting well. Maybe a weight loss clinic, but not a place for researching your particular situation.

Use your health diary to search on the internet for articles that match how you are feeling. Use the test results from your doctor to look things up.

If you cannot find a functional or integrative doctor in your area, expand your search. Most functional doctors don't have to see you. They will send you a health questionnaire and decide what organic tests need to be completed, according to your answers.

Make sure you get a good feeling about the facility. Not all functional doctors are created equally.

- Multiple symptoms that appear to be unrelated are usually diagnosed by Western doctors as caused by depression and anxiety. Not true. When the body goes out of balance, it becomes depressed and anxious.
- Have your hormones checked using a twelve-hour saliva collection test. Hormones change all day long, and a blood sample taken at any given moment is not a true test for hormone imbalances. Hormone imbalances cause so many things. Western world doctors diagnose the symptoms as prescription-needing disease—*not so.*
- Environmental toxins are in all of us. I suggest that everyone who has multiple symptoms that don't seem to be related order a hair analysis to see if heavy metals are present.
- Also, have a trace mineral test done to see if your trace minerals are within the functional medically accepted values. Are some too high? Are some too low? Are some too far out of balance when compared with other minerals? A functional doctor will know what this test says about your body. It all means something. Remember, Clint's hormone doctor was not able to understand the tests that she requested he have taken. His nutritional/functional doctor could.

When your trace minerals levels are not balanced, you are out of
balance, and this causes anxiety, depression, and so many other
unrelated symptoms

Leaky gut can cause so many problems. It is a very good idea to start
there when looking for answers. Inflammation, arthritis,
headaches, exhaustion, and so many other symptoms often are
caused by poor digestion and weak intestines.

It takes a lot of work to give your body what it needs to self-repair. It's
not easy to find a doctor to help you do this. Taking charge of your healthy
choices will empower you to win the battle. Be a health warrior, and seek
the truth.

A final thought

"Hey Doc., this is Sam Neverquestion, I am on the 10th floor of the building that is 3 buildings over from your office. There is a loud ringing in my ears. Shrill, painful can you help me?"

"Ok Sam, I'll send over some ear plugs and drops. That will lessen the sound."

"Hey Doc., this is Sam again. Look my feet are getting hot and tingling. Very painful can you help me? The ear plugs are great, I can't hear that loud ring anymore. Thanks."

"Ok Sam, I'll send over some ice packs, salve and a pair of insulated boots for you to wear. That will stop the burning for sure. Make sure to keep the ear plugs in and keep the boots on. You'll be feeling better in a few days."

"Hey Doc., this is Sam. Sorry but my lungs are congested and I am having trouble breathing. Can you help? The ear plugs and boots are amazing. Wow, I can't thank you enough. But my lungs are very congested and I can't get any air."

"Ok Sam. I'll send over an oxygen tank and mask. You should only need about 2 liters of air for now. You may have to increase in a few hours. How are the ear plugs and boots doing?"

"Hey Doc, Sam here. Listen my lungs are doing much better with the oxygen. I did have to increase the liter dose as you suspected. But now my eyes are blurry and getting very dried out. I can hardly see. It's like smoke in front of me. What can you do?"

"Ok Sam, I will send over some prescription eye drops for dry eyes and a pair of goggles. Keep those on and put the drops in every 5 minutes. How's everything else going? You should be feeling pretty good. I'm taking very good care of you. Oh, by the way, I need your insurance information."

"Hey Doc., this is ummmm Sam, yes that's my name, Sam. You know over here on the 10th floor 3 buildings over from your office. The eye drops and goggles are helping. But now I am in so much pain. Hot. I bet my temperature is at least 125 degrees if not 500 degrees. I'm just too hot to know for sure and feeling scared and anxious like maybe we are missing something. Can you help?"

"OK Sam, you probably need an antibiotic and some pain meds. Not sure what's going on but take the pills per the prescription and you will feel better in a little while."

"Hey Doc., I can hardly speak. My head is dizzy, my feet are on fire, my lungs burn and I cannot see. What is wrong?"

"Ok Sam, you have depression and anxiety. Not sure why. But, it happens. I'll send over some gabapentin and Zoloft. Hang in there, you are getting better."

"Hey Doc, I am in serious pain. I mean like 15 to 20 on that pain scale you doctor's use. I hurt everywhere. I am doing everything you are telling me to do."

"OK Sam, I will send over some Oxycodone. It will stop your pain. Let me know how you are doing."

"Hey Doc., this is Fire Chief Roger, can you please come over to the 3rd building south of yours? I believe we have found a patient of yours that burned to death and fell 10 stories to his death. I believe you were treating him for everything except the obvious. The building was on fire.”

“Ok Chief, I am on my way. But you know he was severely depressed and had many medical issues. I am sure he overdosed on his meds. I told him to take them exactly as prescribed. You know how these drug dependent people are.”

About the Author

Margaret Starr has three children, one of whom suffered from a devastating illness.

Tiltissues@outlook.com

www.ingramcontent.com/pod-product-compliance
Lightning Source LLC
Chambersburg PA
CBHW051439250726
48655CB00001B/140